PRESCRIPTION

or **POISON?**

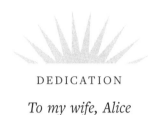

DEDICATION

To my wife, Alice

Ordering

Trade bookstores in the U.S. and Canada please contact:

Publishers Group West
1700 Fourth Street, Berkeley CA 94710
Phone: (800) 788-3123   Fax: (800) 351-5073

Hunter House books are available at bulk discounts for textbook course adoptions;
to qualifying community, health-care, and government organizations;
and for special promotions and fund-raising. For details please contact:

Special Sales Department
Hunter House Inc., PO Box 2914, Alameda CA 94501-0914
Phone: (510) 865-5282   Fax: (510) 865-4295
E-mail: ordering@hunterhouse.com

Individuals can order our books from most bookstores,
by calling (**800**) **266-5592**, or from our website at
www.hunterhouse.com

PRESCRIPTION

or POISON?

The Benefits
and Dangers
of Herbal
Remedies

AMITAVA DASGUPTA, PhD

Hunter House PUBLISHERS

Hunter House Inc., Publishers
PO Box 2914
Alameda CA 94501-0914

Library of Congress Cataloging-in-Publication Data
Dasgupta, Amitava, 1958-
Prescription or poison? : the benefits and dangers of herbal remedies / Amitava Dasgupta.
p.   cm.
Includes bibliographical references and index.
ISBN 978-0-89793-550-0 (trade paper)
1. Herbs—Toxicology.   2. Herbs—Therapeutic use.   I. Title.
RA1250.D37 2009
615'.321—dc22   2009024808

Project Credits

Cover Design	Brian Dittmar Design, Inc.
Book Production	John McKercher
Copy Editor	Margaret Wimberger
Proofreader	John David Marion
Indexer	Nancy D. Peterson
Managing Editor	Alexandra Mummery
Editorial Intern	Ashley Zeal
Senior Marketing Associate	Reina Santana
Publicity Associate	Sean Harvey
Rights Coordinator	Candace Groskreutz
Customer Service Manager	Christina Sverdrup
Order Fulfillment	Washul Lakdhon
Administrator	Theresa Nelson
Computer Support	Peter Eichelberger
Publisher	Kiran S. Rana

Printed and Bound by Bang Printing, Brainerd, Minnesota
Manufactured in the United States of America

9 8 7 6 5 4 3 2 1   First Edition   10 11 12 13 14

Contents

Important Note

The material in this book is intended to provide a review of information regarding the efficacy and toxicity of herbal remedies, as well as the interrelations between herbal supplements and Western drugs. Every effort has been made to provide accurate and dependable information. The contents of this book have been compiled through professional research and in consultation with medical and mental-health professionals. However, health-care professionals have differing opinions, and advances in medical and scientific research are made very quickly, so some of the information may become outdated.

Therefore, the publisher, authors, and editors, as well as the professionals quoted in the book, cannot be held responsible for any error, omission, or dated material. The authors and publisher assume no responsibility for any outcome of applying the information in this book in a program of self-care or under the care of a licensed practitioner. If you have questions concerning your nutrition or diet, or about the application of the information described in this book, consult a qualified health-care professional.

A Note on Usage

Throughout the book generic drug names are used, but occasionally trade names for well-known drugs are included in parenthesis to help ground the nonmedical reader. A full listing of generic and trade names used in this book appears in Appendix A.

Preface

Today, a significant percentage of Americans turn to complementary and alternative medicines to improve their health. These medicines include herbal remedies, traditional Chinese medicines, Ayurvedic medicines, and homeopathic remedies as well as noninvasive modalities such as massage, energy work, yoga, acupuncture, and meditation. In general, people who use these alternative therapies have a college degree and a decent income; also, more women than men use alternative therapies. People turn to complementary and alternative medicine thinking that such therapies are safe and effective and are a viable alternative to Western medicine. Although many alternative modalities such as energy work, massage, yoga, and meditation are safe and may also have efficacy, not all herbal remedies are safe. Because of a general misconception that anything "natural" is safe, people use herbal remedies based on recommendations from friends, family members, or store clerks who might not be educated in medicine or pharmacology. Many users of herbal remedies suffer ill effects. Many books, readily available in health-food stores and bookstores, focus on the efficacy of a variety of herbal supplements with little discussion of toxicity, drug-herb interaction, and food-drug interaction. In addition, these books are mostly based on the personal experience of the authors rather than published information in medical literature.

In this book, I present an unbiased view of the benefits and dangers of herbal remedies based on published articles in the medical literature as well as results published by our research group on herbal remedies. In Chapter 1, I discuss the demographics of people who use complementary and alternative medicine and the most popular herbal remedies in the United States. In Chapter 2, some safe and effective herbs are discussed. At present, scientific research shows that approximately fifty herbs are relatively safe, and some of them are also effective. Chapter 3 is dedicated to a discussion of essential oils and fish oils. Many essential oils have antibacterial properties, and tea tree oil is effective in treating minor skin rashes. Lavender oil has a soothing effect, and massage using essential oil has health benefits. Eating fish or taking fish oil supplements also has certain health benefits. In Chapter 4, herbal remedies that may boost the immune system are discussed. Echinacea is a safe herb and may be effective in reducing symptoms from flu and cold. Chapter 5 is dedicated to a discussion of homeopathic remedies. Although how homeopathy works cannot be explained with modern scientific theory, the efficacy of certain homeopathic remedies has been published in the medical literature. In addition, adverse effects from the use of homeopathic remedies are rare. In Chapter 6, vitamin and mineral supplements are discussed. Contrary to popular belief, vitamins in megadoses are toxic and excess intake of fat-soluble vitamins such as vitamins D, A, K, and E may increase mortality rather than prolong healthy life. For a healthy person, one multivitamin/mineral supplement a day is sufficient. However, pregnant women may need more folate and iron, and the elderly must also take multivitamin/multimineral supplements based on the recommendation of their physicians. Chapters 7 and 8 discuss herbal supplements that may cause organ damage, toxicity, and even death. In Chapter 9, I discuss herbal remedies that interact with Western drugs, causing toxicity. At the end of the book, trade names of all these drugs are listed for easy reference. Certain medications also interact with your food and drink. If you are taking certain medications for treating a chronic condition, you should consult with your doctor to see if you can drink grapefruit juice. Chapter 10 discusses drug-food interactions. Chapter 11 specifically addresses herbs used by women, while Chapter 12 covers the effects herbal medicines can have on the results of clinical laboratory tests. In Chapter 13, herbal medicines contaminated with lead and other toxic metals are discussed. Chapter 14 is devoted to discussion of Ayurvedic medicines, some of which contain heavy metals such as lead, arsenic, and mercury, either as a component or as a contaminant. Some traditional Chinese medicines produced in China and Hong Kong are contaminated with heavy metals or Western drugs. Consumers should be aware of taking such contaminated products.

Currently, there is a lot of enthusiasm among doctors, pharmacists, and scientists regarding herbal medicines because it is possible to isolate their active components, and these might be the drugs of the future. Many medical-school curriculums incorporate herbal medicine. Your doctor, nurse, and pharmacist should be knowledgeable about herbal remedies, and disclosing the remedies you are taking to your doctor is a good idea because he or she can likely guide you to avoid unwanted herbal supplements and take the ones which may help you. Your doctors, nurses, and pharmacists are committed to what is best for your health, and a holistic approach to treatment is sometimes useful. Like many physicians and scientists, I have received grants from pharmaceutical industries for conducting research, but none of us sell our souls to the pharmaceutical industry. It is not true that doctors are against complementary and alternative medicines because they are loyal to the pharmaceutical industries. Your doctor is committed to your well-being and your health. Certain herbal remedies may do more harm than good, and when your doctor asks you to stop taking such a supplement, he or she is looking at what is best for you and nothing else. Therefore, trust your doctor and disclose all herbal supplements you are taking. You will be glad that you did.

Acknowledgments

I would like to thank Jacqueline G. Garcia, MBA, EdD, for critically reading and editing the entire manuscript and providing helpful suggestions. Ms. Alice Wells also read the entire manuscript, and I thank her for her helpful comments. Last but not least, I thank my wife, Alice, for putting up with me during the long evening and weekend hours I devoted to writing this book.

— Amitava Dasgupta, PhD
Houston, Texas

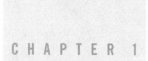

CHAPTER 1

Complementary and Alternative Medicines: Who Uses Them?

For most of human history, herbal remedies were the only medicines available to treat various illnesses. About one hundred years ago, 59 percent of all medicines listed in the 1890 version of the U.S. Pharmacopeia were from herbal products.[1] Today, as many as one-third to approximately one-half of all drugs on the market are derived from plants or natural sources. For example, the antibiotic streptomycin is derived from a soil bacterium (*Streptomyces griseus*), while the immunosuppressant drug cyclosporine, which is used to prevent organ rejection in transplant recipients, is derived from a soil fungus. Several anticancer drugs, such as vincristine, vinblastine, and paclitaxel (Taxol), are also derived from plants. The widely used cardioactive drug digoxin is extracted from the foxglove plant (*Digitalis lanata*). So, the question is: Since herbal supplements are derived from plants, do we need to exercise caution in taking them in the same way we take precautions when using prescription drugs?

> **Myth: Anything natural is safe.**
> **Reality: Some natural products are safe, but others can be toxic.**

This book is an honest discussion of the benefits and dangers of herbal remedies and is based on published reports in medical journals.

The major differences between natural supplements and Western drugs are as follows:

1. When Western drugs are prepared from plants, specific manufacturing processes are employed to isolate the active natural ingredient from other

crude plant products. In addition, rigorous quality-control procedures are in place to ensure that the amount of the active ingredient is constant or nearly consistent among all samples. So if you take one digoxin tablet containing 0.6 mg of digoxin today and you take another digoxin tablet six months later from a different prescription refill, you will ingest the same amount of digoxin. In the preparation of herbal supplements, such rigorous quality-control procedures are not always adhered to. For example, in different St.-John's-wort preparations, the amount of the active ingredients may vary widely.

2. There is a big difference between taking crude natural products and the Western drugs prepared from them. Are you willing to eat fungus instead of taking a penicillin-containing antibiotic tablet in which the penicillin is derived from fungus? Think about another scenario. Can you run your car on crude oil? Not only must oil be refined first, but some manufacturers recommend that you use premium gasoline in your car. Many herbal supplements can be used as a starting material for future drugs, but just as oil needs refining and grapes need fermenting, natural active ingredients need to be isolated from the plant before they can be used as medicines.

3. Many plant products are toxic. When a tiger is on the prowl, a gazelle runs for its life. Unfortunately, plants can't run away from danger. Therefore, they produce toxic substances to discourage animals from eating them. Frequently, these products are toxic to humans as well. In an herbal supplement, one ingredient might produce the desired therapeutic benefit, while other ingredients produce toxicity. Since all components are extracted together in making herbal supplements and good components are not usually separated from toxic components, toxicity may occur following the use of common herbal supplements.

4. Western medicines may also cause toxicity, but due to rigorous research, these toxic effects quickly become known to health-care providers. Toxicities of herbal supplements are not well studied. For example, during the 1990s, kava, an herbal supplement used as an antianxiety and sleep aid, was considered relatively safe and as effective as tricyclic antidepressants. However, now it is well established that long-term use of kava may cause severe liver toxicity and even death. It is interesting that the South Pacific Islanders who use kava drinks for religious ceremonies do not suffer from

kava-induced liver toxicity. This may be due to the fact that they drink kava extract infrequently or they drink aqueous (water) extract of kava, which may not contain harmful chemicals. Most kava products sold in the United States are a water/alcohol extract of the plant.

5. Some herbalists argue that herbal remedies were used for thousands of years and that native people reaped the medical benefits and did not experience toxicity. The truth is, native people often chewed leaves or roots or prepared tea by boiling plant parts. Therefore, only small amounts of plant alkaloids (active ingredients as well as toxic substances) were extracted, which may have caused lesser toxicity. In addition, historical documentation of toxicity from herbal remedies may be poor because those native people may not have reported adverse effects out of respect for the healers. Today, herbal supplements are prepared using modern extraction techniques and therefore most likely contain more active ingredients, thus potentially causing more toxicity.

6. One reason some herbal supplements may cause toxicity is the dosage. It is well documented that most drugs are toxic if given in high dosages. Even aspirin and acetaminophen (Tylenol) can kill you if you take too much, and emergency rooms worldwide commonly deal with life-threatening poisoning from these easily available over-the-counter drugs. Acetaminophen, if taken for a long time at a high dosage, can cause significant liver toxicity but is safe at the recommended dosage—a maximum of up to 2,000 mg (2 gm) per day—for a few days. Under a physician's advice even a maximum dosage of up to 4,000 mg per day (4 gm) for a few days is tolerable, but people who consume alcohol may experience liver toxicity even with the lower recommended dosage of acetaminophen. Some popular over-the-counter (OTC) medications might contain acetaminophen under different names, so when combining medications, always make sure that the totals do not exceed the recommended dosage. If you consume alcohol on a daily basis, do not take acetaminophen or acetaminophen-containing medication without consulting a doctor. Do not consume alcohol when you take acetaminophen. Dosages of many herbal supplements are not determined by rigorous clinical trials, and in most cases are determined without any extensive study using human subjects. Toxicities of many herbal supplements such as kava have been documented to be dosage-related.

Just as safe drugs such as aspirin and acetaminophen, if taken at very high dosage, can cause life-threatening toxicity, toxicities of many herbal remedies may be related to high dosage.

Is Any Herbal Remedy Safe?

Of course, many herbal supplements are safe, as are several plant oils intended for topical use to treat local infection, skin rashes, and related problems. Tea-tree oil and eucalyptus oil have antibacterial properties and are a safe and effective way to treat a skin rash. However, if a rash does not resolve in four to seven days, you may need to contact a health-care provider. Green tea and various herbal teas such as ginseng tea are safe and can be used as health tonics. According to the authors of one published report, comfrey, life root, borage, calamus, chaparral, licorice, and Ma Huang are unsafe; relatively safe herbs include feverfew, garlic, ginkgo, Asian ginseng, saw palmetto, St. John's wort, and valerian.[2]

Does the FDA Control the Sale of Herbal Supplements?

The U.S. Food and Drug Administration (FDA) regulates all prescription and non-prescription drugs sold in the United States. For example, phenylpropanolamine, a common ingredient of many over-the-counter cold medications, is no longer approved for use because it may cause toxicity to the heart. Within a few weeks following the FDA ban, all drug manufacturers withdrew cold medications containing phenylpropanolamine and replaced that active ingredient with a safer alternative. Herbal remedies are sold under the 1994 Dietary Supplement Health and Education Act and are classified as food supplements. According to this law, food supplements also include vitamins, minerals, amino acids, extracts, metabolites, etc. Manufacturers of herbal remedies are not allowed to claim any medical benefit from using their products, but they are not under surveillance by the FDA. Therefore, unlike drugs, dietary supplements can be manufactured and sold without demonstrating safety and efficacy to the FDA.

For a new drug, the manufacturer must demonstrate the safety and efficacy to the FDA before the drug can be sold legally in the United States. In contrast, for herbal remedies, the FDA has the burden to prove that a supplement is unsafe and/or to recommend that the product be removed from the market. Unfortunately, even after recommending that an herbal supplement is not safe and should be withdrawn from the market, the FDA cannot legally force the manufacturer to stop producing or selling that particular product. For example, in 2002 the FDA issued a warning regarding the safety of kava because it had been reported that prolonged use of kava could cause serious liver damage. However, even today, kava products are widely available in health-food stores. The Canadian government also issued warnings against the use of kava, but two months after the advisory, twenty-two of thirty-four stores surveyed in Toronto recommended the use of kava and only nine mentioned any safety concerns. The authors in this Canadian study concluded that federal advisories may not affect the sales of unsafe products.[3]

In many countries, herbal supplements are not well regulated. However, in 1978 Germany created an expert committee, called Committee E, to review herbal drugs and preparations from medicinal plants. Committee E issued a series of monographs on the safety and efficacy of herbal products that were based on a review of historical information; chemical, pharmacological, clinical, and toxicological study findings; case reports; epidemiological data; and unpublished manufacturers' data. If an herb has an approved monograph, it can be marketed. (All 380 Commission E monographs are collected in book form; the commission no longer exists.) Currently, there is a push for streamlining regulation of the European market for herbal supplements. A directive released in 2004 by the European Parliament and the Council of Europe now provides the basis for regulation of herbal supplements in European markets. This directive requires that herbal medicines be authorized by the national regulatory authorities of each European country and that these products must be safe. The safety of a supplement will be established based on published scientific literature, and when safety is not deemed sufficient, it will be communicated to consumers. In Europe, there will be two kinds of herbal supplements in the future: herbal supplements with well-established safety and efficacy, and traditional herbal supplements, which do not have a recognized level of efficacy but are deemed to be relatively safe.[4]

The Australian government created the Complementary Medicines Evaluation Committee in 1997 to address regulatory issues regarding herbal remedies. The Canadian government implemented a policy on 1 January 2004 to regulate natural health products. Naturopaths, traditional Chinese-medicine practitioners, homeopaths, and herbalists in Canada are concerned that this policy will eventually affect their access to the products they need to practice effectively.[5]

The Sale of Herbal Supplements Is on the Rise

In the United States, the sale of herbal remedies skyrocketed from $200 million in 1988 to over $3.3 billion in 1997; to an estimated $15.7 billion a mere three years later, in 2000; and to an estimated $18.8 billion in 2003.[6] The use of herbal remedies is also widespread in the European Community, with an estimated annual sale of $7 billion in 2001.[7] It is estimated that roughly 20,000 herbal products are available in the United States, and in one survey, approximately one out of five adults reported using an herbal supplement within the past year. The ten most commonly used herbal supplements are echinacea, ginseng, ginkgo biloba, garlic, St. John's wort, peppermint, ginger, soy, chamomile, and kava.[8]

Complementary and Alternative Medicines

Complementary and alternative medicines (CAM) include naturopathy, homeopathy, herbal supplements, traditional Chinese medicines, Indian Ayurvedic medicines, diet-based therapy, chiropractic, massage therapy, Reiki and other types of energy healing, acupuncture, yoga, biofeedback, hypnosis, meditation, and prayer. The use of the many modalities of CAM is on the rise in the United States and in many other countries around the world. In addition, people are also becoming increasingly interested in consuming organic food and following healthy diets. Although this book is focused on herbal remedies, a brief discussion of other types of complementary and alternative therapies may be helpful.

Many people approach CAM practitioners to address problems such as chronic pain and fatigue when there is a perception that these problems are not adequately addressed by their primary-care physician. A large number of people also believe that natural remedies are much safer than Western drugs. In addition, pseudo-medical jargon and elaborate marketing claims confuse many consumers and encourage them to believe in the efficacy of unproven alternative therapies.[9] In Table 1.1, the estimated number of people using various types of CAM in 1999 and 2002 are listed.[10] In 2002 the most commonly used CAM in the United States was herbal supplements, which were taken by an estimated 38 million adults, followed by relaxation techniques (29 million adults) and chiropractic (15 million adults). Among CAM users, 41 percent used two or more CAM therapies.[11]

TABLE 1.1: Estimated U.S. Population Using Various Types of Complementary and Alternative Medicine in 1999 and 2002

CAM THERAPY	ESTIMATED POPULATION	
	1999*	2002[†]
Spiritual healing/prayer	26,997,000	No data
Herbal supplements	18,937,000	38,183,000
Relaxation therapy	9,891,000	29,220,000
Chiropractic	14,969,000	15,226,000
Yoga	No data	10,386,000
Homeopathy	6,182,000	3,433,000
Acupuncture	2,691,000	2,136,000
Energy healing/Reiki	2,142,000	1,080,000
Hypnosis	1,013,000	505,000
Biofeedback	1,029,000	278,000

* Estimated number based on data published by Ni et al.[12]

[†] Estimated number based on data published by Tindle et al.[13] The authors estimated these numbers using 2002 National Health Interview Survey (31,044 respondents) and then using complex statistical analysis using a U.S. adult population of 205,825,095.

These studies give the latest comprehensive data available. Osteopathic medicine is not included because doctors in osteopathic medicine are licensed, just like MDs. Dietary and nutritional supplement use was not studied.

The Benefits of Massage, Reiki, and Other Bio-Field Therapies

The National Center for Complementary and Alternative Medicine classifies therapeutic touch, healing touch, and Reiki as bio-field therapies and acknowledges the use of such subtle energy therapies for health benefits. These therapies are noninvasive and are based on compassionate touch and the presence of a provider who is willing to help the recipient. They take place in a calm and nurturing environment, in contrast to the traditional stressful environment of medical therapies. Healing-touch practices are found throughout the history of nursing, and the American Holistic Nurses Association endorses energy therapies.[14]

Noninvasive CAM can be fairly safe if the practitioner is properly trained. For example, massage therapy can provide relaxation and other benefits and is best if performed by a licensed massage therapist who has undergone extensive training procedures and who understands for which diseases or conditions massage therapy is not appropriate. If you go to an untrained therapist with lower-back pain, the therapy may hurt you more than help you. If you are on a tight budget, consider going to a massage therapy school for treatment; a student therapist may offer treatment at a cost substantially lower than a practicing licensed therapist. Massage therapy is offered at several cancer centers in the United States, and medical researchers have proven the effectiveness of massage therapy in reducing anxiety, pain, and other symptoms in cancer patients.[15]

According to a British report, the six most commonly used complementary therapies there are reflexology, massage, yoga, relaxation and meditation, acupuncture, and aromatherapy. These therapies have been shown to benefit people suffering from multiple sclerosis.[16] In one clinical trial, the authors concluded that reflexology may have a positive effect in alleviating lower-back pain.[17] Tai chi, acupuncture, acupressure, yoga, and meditation have improved sleep patterns in older adults in a limited number of early trials.[18] Interestingly, these types of therapies are also gaining popularity in the United States.

Reiki, which originated in Japan, is an energy-based touch therapy used to balance life force (chi). This therapy is based on the Eastern belief that the body needs a continuous flow of life force in order to maintain health and well-being. There are even practitioners who perform Reiki on pets. If you wish to experience Reiki healing, please visit a Reiki master, a practitioner who has undergone formal training and can also advise you whether you need to see a medical doctor for your condition. The medical literature is divided on whether Reiki can really help or not. Some research clearly indicates the benefits of Reiki healing, while other reports fail to show a statistically significant benefit in patient groups receiving Reiki healing versus patients who did not. Nevertheless, to this author's knowledge there is no report that demonstrates any harmful effect of Reiki, massage, or any other form of bio-field therapy.

> *Massage therapy, Reiki, reflexology, and other bio-field therapies may be beneficial, but please see a licensed or otherwise qualified practitioner. Going to an untrained or self-claimed practitioner may cause more harm than good.*

The Benefits of Acupuncture

Acupuncture, part of traditional Chinese medicine, is an invasive technique in which fine needles are inserted into specific points of the body for therapeutic benefits. According to Chinese theory, acupuncture points lie along meridians through which the body's vital energy, chi (qi), flows. There is no known anatomical basis of this theory in modern medicine. Because acupuncture is an invasive technique, it is not free from adverse effects. However, risk from acupuncture is low if practiced by a trained professional who uses sterile, disposable needles. Scientific research has indicated that acupuncture appears to be effective in alleviating postoperative nausea and vomiting, chemotherapy-associated nausea and vomiting, postoperative dental pain, migraine headaches, and lower-back pain. For conditions such as fibromyalgia, osteoarthritis of the knee, and tennis elbow, acupuncture appears to have promising results. But for conditions such as drug addiction, other chronic pain, neck pain, and asthma, the results are inconclusive. For smoking cessation, tinnitus, and weight loss, the evidence that acupuncture is beneficial is usually regarded as negative.[19] In one report, the authors synthesized results from thirty-three scientific studies using meta-analysis and concluded that although it is not more effective than other therapies, acupuncture effectively decreases chronic lower-back pain.[20] Another study concluded that short-term abdominal acupuncture is more effective than medication in relieving insomnia in women. In addition, acupuncture has few adverse effects.[21]

The Benefits of Yoga, Meditation, and Prayer

Yoga originated in ancient India; it is a Sanskrit word that means "disciplining or aligning mind and body for spiritual growth." Yoga includes a variety of techniques including postures (*asanas*) and breathing exercises (*pranayama*), and it may include the chanting of mantras, changes in lifestyle, and the incorporation of spiritual beliefs and rituals. It is estimated that in 2002 approximately 10.4 million adults in the United States were practicing yoga; the majority of these people were Caucasians (85 percent), females (76 percent), and college-educated; the mean age was thirty-nine. A majority of yoga users (61 percent) felt yoga was important in maintaining health.[22] Yoga improved exercise tolerance and positively affected markers of inflammation in serum (C-reactive protein, interleukin-6) in patients with heart failure. In addition, yoga also improved quality of life in these patients.[23] Yoga may also be effective in controlling blood pressure, managing secondary complications due to chronic hypertension, and reducing stress. In addition, yoga may lower cholesterol, though the mechanism is unknown, and it may be beneficial as an adjunct therapy for patients suffering from non-insulin-dependent diabetes. Yoga also aids the recovery process after a heart attack (myocardial infarction), and it generally improves quality of life.[24] However, there is one adverse reaction reported in a woman who developed thrombosis. This was attributed to adopting an unusual neck posture during yoga practice.[25]

Meditation may be effective for patients coping with medical and psychological problems.

Benefits of meditation, prayer, yoga, and relaxation therapy were observed in patients with epilepsy, anxiety disorders, and nonpsychiatric mood disorders. In addition, these techniques are also effective in reducing symptoms of premenstrual discomfort, menopause, and autoimmune illness. Meditation also improves mood in cancer patients.[26]

Surveys indicate that the majority of patients in the United States have spiritual beliefs, and during illness greater spiritual need may arise. Many scientific studies suggest that religious belief and spirituality are linked with better clinical outcomes, increased life span, improved coping skills, and even higher health-related quality of life during terminal illness. In addition, spiritual beliefs are associated with decreased anxiety, depression, and risk of suicide.[27] Spiritual advisors are available to both patients and health-care providers in the majority of hospitals in North America. Cotton et al. reported that spirituality and religious decision-making were positively correlated with health outcomes in the adolescent population.[28] In another report, the author found a strong relationship between prayer and the well-being of breast cancer survivors and commented that health-care providers should encourage women diagnosed with breast cancer to explore their spirituality as an effective resource for coping with physical and psychological responses to cancer.[29]

Mind-body therapies such as yoga, meditation, spirituality, and prayer are beneficial for improving quality of life and reducing stress for healthy individuals. These therapies may also benefit patients recovering from various illnesses.

Who Takes Herbal Supplements?

Between 1990 and 1997 the estimated number of visits to complementary and alternative-medicine practitioners increased by 47 percent (425 million visits to practitioners in 1990 versus 629 million in 1997.) In 1997 an estimated 34 percent of U.S. adults were using complementary and alternative medicines, and in 2002 a 25 percent increase was observed. The highest percentage of users of complementary and alternative medicines were female, were between the ages of forty and sixty-four, were non-black/non-Hispanic, and had an average annual income of $65,000 or higher. While use of herbal supplements and yoga increased steadily between 1997 and 2002, that of other therapies remained stable or decreased.[30] Another study estimated that 28.9 percent of U.S. adults used at least one form of complementary or alternative therapy during the previous year and that use of such therapy was most prevalent among women between thirty-five and fifty-four years of age. The overall use of such therapies was higher in white non-Hispanic persons than in Hispanic and black non-Hispanic persons, and use of complementary and alternative therapies was higher among individuals in good health. Interestingly, people who use such therapies were also more likely to consult conventional medical services.[31]

> *In general, more women than men use complementary and alternative medicines.*

Use of herbal remedies is generally higher among Asians and Pacific Islanders living in the United States than among non-Hispanic whites. A study found that use of herbal supplements in Asians and Pacific Islanders living in the United States is higher among women sixty or older and among people who have more education and/or higher incomes. The same study also found that 44 percent of the Chinese Americans surveyed reported use of herbal supplements.[32]

Individuals with illnesses tend to use herbal supplements more than healthy people. The use of complementary and alternative medicines is very common among patients infected with HIV. In general, approximately 42 percent of participants in a nationwide survey indicate use of complementary and alternative medicines, but among patients infected with HIV, this percentage can be as high as 80 percent. Reasons cited by these patients for using alternative therapies include expectation of a cure, reduction of disease or of side effects from medications, desire to have more control over the disease process, and improvement in quality of life. The therapies used by these patients include megavitamins, herbal supplements, lifestyle and exercise changes, diet, counseling, and prayer.[33] The highly active antiretroviral therapy (HAART), which uses a cocktail of several drugs including newer protease inhibitors, is very useful in controlling viral load in patients with the HIV infection. However, nonadherence to HAART is detrimental and causes treatment failure. In addition, there may be potentially serious interactions between herbal supplements and drugs used in HAART. Although adherence to HAART and the use of complementary and alternative medicine in patients infected with HIV is mixed, one recent report indicates that women who use such therapy show decreased adherence to HAART.[34]

Use of complementary and alternative medicines is also common among cancer patients and survivors. In one report, 66 percent of women with breast cancer used at least one alternative therapy during the previous twelve months, and the majority of these patients did not inform their physicians of their use of these alternative therapies. The reason reported for using such therapies was the belief that they could prevent cancer recurrences and/or improve the quality of life.[35]

> *Patients taking antiretroviral drugs for the treatment of HIV should never use herbal supplements without approval of their physicians. Taking vitamin and mineral supplements is okay, but megavitamin therapy may be harmful because excess vitamin C can cause kidney stones, and fat-soluble vitamins (vitamin A, D, E, and K) have toxicity. Please consult your health-care provider before initiating megavitamin therapy.*

Health conditions that lead people to explore alternative therapies include:

- arthritis
- chronic pain
- depression
- fatigue
- HIV
- phobias
- anxiety
- cancer
- diabetes
- headache
- life-threatening or terminal illness
- smoking

- stress
- women's issues (including menstrual problems, urinary tract infection, infertility, nausea and vomiting during pregnancy, and menopausal symptoms)
- organ transplant

Health-Care Providers Using Complementary and Alternative Medicines

There is a general perception that health-care providers do not believe in complementary and alternative medicine because pharmaceutical companies and doctors are afraid that they will lose business. So you might be surprised to learn that health-care providers also use complementary and alternative medicine. I myself use homeopathic remedies for stress control because these remedies have no side effects. In one survey of 1,249 health-care professionals, 51 percent reported using herbal supplements; use was higher among physicians' assistants and nurse practitioners (63 percent), clinical nurses (59 percent), and medical and nursing students (52 percent). According to this survey, 48 percent of physicians, 40 percent of dietitians, and 37 percent of pharmacists also used herbal supplements.[36]

Common Herbal Supplements Taken by American Adults

Any herbal supplement, such as St. John's wort, that has many reported interactions with medications should be avoided if prescription medication is being taken—especially for controlling a chronic condition. Among the herbal products used by American adults, the most common was echinacea (41 percent). The other herbal supplements used by respondents in that study include ginseng (25 percent), ginkgo biloba (22 percent), garlic (20 percent), St. John's wort (12.2 percent), peppermint (12 percent), and ginger (10.5 percent). The estimated U.S. population taking various herbal supplements according to this report is summarized in Table 1.2 on the next page. The most common condition for the use of herbal supplements among people who use them was head or chest colds (30 percent), followed by musculoskeletal conditions (16 percent) and stomach or intestinal problems (11 percent). The authors of this study found that the majority of people who use herbal supplements were between the ages of twenty-five and forty-four.[37]

TABLE 1.2: Estimated U.S. Population Taking Various Herbal Supplements

HERBAL SUPPLEMENT	ESTIMATED POPULATION	INDICATION FOR USE
Echinacea	14,665,000	Boosting immune system (avoiding cold, flu)
Ginseng	8,777,000	Tonic for general well-being
Ginkgo biloba	7,679,000	Dementia
Garlic	7,096,000	Lowering cholesterol
St. John's wort	4,390,000	Depression
Peppermint	4,308,000	Nausea and vomiting
Ginger	3,768,000	Nausea and vomiting
Soy	3,480,000	High cholesterol, high blood pressure, menopausal symptoms
Kava*	2,441,000	Anxiety
Valerian	2,131,000	Sedative
Saw palmetto	2,054,000	Prostate conditions
Evening primrose	1,686,000	Eczema, inflammation
Black cohosh	1,510,000	Symptoms of menopause
Ma Huang (ephedra)*	1,474,000	Weight-loss aid
Licorice	1,469,000	Adrenal-gland support (cortisol) and multiple other uses
Milk thistle	1,255,000	Liver dysfunction
Guarana	1,085,000	Energy booster
Comfrey*	938,000	Local use for broken bones
Dong Quai	815,000	Symptoms of menopause
Hawthorn	733,000	Tonic for cardiac health
Cascara sagrada	663,000	Laxative
Bladderwrack/kelp	497,000	Underactive thyroid
Chaparral*	246,000	Autoimmune disease and allergy

Estimated number of people taking any herbal supplement was calculated using complicated statistical techniques based on reports of the National Health Interview Survey (2002) and an estimate of the U.S. population from the Census Bureau.

* This is a very toxic herb that should be avoided at all costs.

Both users and nonusers of prescription medications take herbal supplements. Of the 31,044 respondents to a National Health Interview Survey in 2002, 67 percent used prescription medication in the prior twelve months; 21 percent of those people used dietary supplements. In addition, of all respondents who used prescription medications and dietary supplements, 69 percent did not disclose their use of dietary supplements to their physicians. Among prescription-medication users, menopausal women (33 percent), those with chronic gastrointestinal disorders (28 percent), and severe-headache sufferers (28 percent) had the highest use of dietary supplements, while people with congestive heart failure (12 percent) and those with a history of coronary artery disease (12 percent) had a lower use.[38] Dietary supplements used by prescription medication users are listed in Table 1.3.

TABLE 1.3: Herbal Dietary Supplements Commonly Used by Prescription-Medication Users

DIETARY SUPPLEMENT	PERCENTAGE OF USERS (%)	INDICATION FOR USE
Echinacea	40.6	Boosting immune system
Ginseng	22.6	Tonic for general well-being
Ginkgo biloba	20.5	Dementia
Garlic	19.4	High cholesterol
Glucosamine/chondroitin	16.0	Osteoarthritis
Black cohosh	13.0	Symptoms of menopause
St. John's wort	12.3	Depression
Peppermint	11.5	Nausea and vomiting
Fish oil	11.2	Omega-3 fatty acids/lowering risk of heart disease
Ginger	10.5	Nausea and vomiting
Soy	10.1	High cholesterol, high blood pressure, and multiple other uses
Ragweed/chamomile	8.7	Sleeplessness and anxiety
Bee pollen	6.7	General health tonic
Kava*	6.4	Anxiety
Valerian	6.1	Anxiety
Saw palmetto	5.7	Prostate conditions
Melatonin	5.2	Insomnia
Evening primrose	4.3	Eczema, inflammation
Licorice	3.9	Adrenal-gland support (cortisol) and multiple other uses
Ma Huang (ephedra)*	3.8	Weight loss
Milk thistle	3.5	Liver dysfunction

* This is a very toxic herb that should be avoided at all costs.

Patients with HIV also use herbal supplements on a widespread basis. According to one report, the most commonly used remedies in these patients are vitamin C (63 percent), multivitamin and mineral supplements (54 percent), vitamin E (53 percent), and garlic (53 percent).[39]

Herbal Remedies and Medical Research

As mentioned earlier, many Western drugs today are derived from plant and natural sources. Pharmaceutical companies and the medical-research community believe that new drugs can be developed from herbal and traditional Chinese medicine, and extensive research is going on in this field. The National Institutes of Health (NIH), an agency of the United States Department of Health and Human Services, is the primary health-care–related research organization of the federal government and the major provider of funding for health-care–related research in the country. The National Center for Complementary and Alternative Medicine (NCCAM) was established in 1991 as the Office of Alternative Medicine and was reorganized and renamed as the NCCAM in 1998. One of the twenty-seven institutes of the NIH, NCCAM is dedicated to exploring complementary and alternative medicines in the context of rigorous scientific research with the goal of developing innovative therapies. The institute also provides grants to researchers for investigating complementary and alternative medicine, and it funds clinical trials to determine their efficacy. The NCCAM's website provides a wealth of information, including updates on recent important scientific discoveries regarding alternative therapies and monographs on many popular herbal supplements. I recommend that anyone interested in pursuing complementary and alternative medicines check the Institute's website for information.

NCCAM—National Institutes of Health
9000 Rockville Pike, Bethesda MD 20892
E-mail: info@nccam.nih.gov   Website: http://nccam.nih.gov

A number of leading medical schools in the United States also have centers for CAM research. Harvard, Columbia, Johns Hopkins, and Stanford have the leading university-based research institutes focusing exclusively on complementary and alternative medicines. In addition, many medical schools, including the one where this author teaches, now offer formal coursework in the field. Several private research organizations are also actively involved in scientific research in CAM, with the goal of improving quality of life for patients and all people.

Conclusion

One-third to one-half of all Western medicines are derived from plants, and there is a strong possibility of finding effective new therapies from the natural environment. Certain herbal supplements have efficacy, but severe toxicities have also been reported following the use of herbal supplements. In contrast, noninvasive complementary and alternative therapies such as massage therapy, energy healing, Reiki and other bio-field therapies, yoga, meditation, and prayer are safe and effective. In addition, invasive therapy such as acupuncture is also relatively safe if practiced by an experienced professional. There are many safe supplements, and if you would like to use them, this book will familiarize you with them. Your doctor, nurse, pharmacist, and other health-care professionals usually have a wealth of knowledge on complementary and alternative therapies, and they may help you find the right practitioner. Homeopathic remedies are also safe.

CHAPTER 2

Some Relatively Safe and Effective Herbal Supplements

Of the many herbal remedies commercially available, about thirty or so different herbal products are commonly used by most Americans. One study found that adults between the ages of forty-five and sixty-four most frequently used herbal supplements, and the most commonly used supplement among these people was echinacea (41 percent). Other frequently used supplements were ginseng (25 percent), ginkgo (22 percent), and garlic (20 percent).[1] Another study reported that the most commonly used herbal supplements in the United States are garlic, ginkgo biloba, echinacea, soy, saw palmetto, ginseng, and St. John's wort.[2] Interestingly, all these herbal supplements are safe and have proven efficacy. St. John's wort, however, should not be used by people taking medications for a chronic condition without permission from their doctor, because it reduces the efficacy of many drugs (see Chapter 9). Herbal remedies may be classified in one of four categories: safe and effective, safe but efficacy has not been proven, borderline safe, and unsafe.

There are several safe and effective herbs that can boost the immune system. These are discussed in detail in Chapter 4. In Chapter 11, herbal supplements that may be beneficial to women are discussed. Table 2.1 lists a variety of conditions and the herbal and nutritional supplements used to treat them.

Generally Recognized as Safe (GRAS) Herbal Supplements

Herbal supplements are sold in the United States under the 1994 Dietary Supplement Health and Education Act. However, just removing the therapeutic-benefit

TABLE 2.1: Commonly Used Herbal and Nutritional Supplements and the Conditions They're Used For

CONDITION	COMMONLY USED HERBS
Anxiety/depression	Chamomile, St. John's wort
Arthritis	Burdock, cat's claw, dandelion, fish oil
Acute/chronic pain	Capsicum, noni
Anticancer	Burdock, green tea, lycopene
Aphrodisiac	Damiana
Benign prostatic hypertrophy (BPH)	Saw palmetto
Cold/sore throat	Astragalus, echinacea, goldenseal, licorice, osha
Constipation	Cascara sagrada, flaxseed, senna
Diabetes	Fenugreek, ginseng, grape seed
Diarrhea/digestive problems	Bilberry, chamomile, dandelion, fennel, green tea
Fatigue	Ginseng, vitamins
General well-being	Minerals, vitamins
High cholesterol	Fenugreek, garlic, grape seed, red clover, fish oil
Insomnia	Valerian
Liver disease/hepatitis	Dandelion, milk thistle, peppermint
Migraine headache	Feverfew
Obesity/overweight	Bitter orange, green tea
Poor blood circulation	Ginkgo biloba, horse chestnut
Weak immune system	Astragalus, cat's claw, echinacea, goldenseal, osha
Women's health issues	Black cohosh, chasteberry, cranberry, Dong Quai, red clover
Wounds/burns/skin problems	Aloe vera, arnica, lavender, lemon balm, turmeric

claim from an herbal supplement may not make it a food. The FDA is trying to control the safety of such dietary supplements by using GRAS status for new supplements after evaluating the safety record provided by the manufacturer. GRAS stands for "generally recognized as safe," a designation used by the FDA to label a food additive as safe for human consumption. GRAS exemptions are granted for substances that are generally recognized among experts as safe for their intended use either through scientific testing procedures or, for substances that have been used in foods prior to January 1958, on common experience for that use. Many botanicals fall into this category, having been used to flavor foods. Many herbals are included because they were used as components of natural flavoring or used as teas.

The FDA may either grant GRAS status by making no comment on the claim or deny GRAS status if it determines that the herbal supplement does not have an adequate safety record. In this case, the FDA notifies the manufacturer of its decision and cause of action. Many herbal products sold today in the United States fall into a gray zone and do not have GRAS status; for example, flaxseed oil, which is generally considered safe as a laxative, does not have GRAS status. Kava has an FDA warning regarding its safety and, as expected, does not have GRAS status. Therefore, if an herbal supplement does not currently have the GRAS status, that does not necessarily mean it is unsafe to consume. In the remainder of this section, various safe herbal supplements are discussed, along with their promoted uses.

Aloe Vera

Aloe vera (*Aloe barbadensis*) is a plant of the lily family that has been used medicinally for more than five thousand years by Egyptians, Indians, Chinese, and Europeans. Aloe-vera gel is an aqueous extract of the leaf pulp and may contain more than seventy active compounds. Traditionally, aloe vera is used topically for wound healing and treating various skin conditions, and it is believed to have anti-inflammatory, antioxidant, antiaging, and immune-boosting properties.[3] Aloe-vera gel is found in many skin lotions, hand creams, and sunscreens, and is also used as a laxative. Scientific studies have indicated that aloe vera has wound-healing properties and may also be helpful in treating genital herpes and plaque psoriasis (the most common form of psoriasis, in which skin is inflamed, red, and covered with scales, found most commonly on the elbows and knees). Aloe vera is effective in healing first- and second-degree burns but not in protecting skin from radiation-induced injury such as sunburn.

Oral intake of aloe vera may lower blood glucose and cholesterol,[4] but diarrhea caused by the use of aloe vera as a laxative may reduce absorption of many drugs. Because aloe vera may lower blood glucose, diabetic patients taking anti-diabetic medicine or insulin should consult with their doctor before taking aloe vera on a regular basis. One clinical trial indicated that aloe vera taken for four weeks produced a good response in treating active ulcerative colitis (a form of inflammatory bowel disease in which the large intestine is swollen and may have ulceration) and is also safe.[5] Aloe vera is an approved botanical on the GRAS list.

Astragalus

Traditionally, astragalus has been used in Chinese medicine in combination with other herbs for boosting the immune system. It is also used in treating the common cold and flu and as a heart tonic. Astragalus is discussed in more detail in Chapter 4.

Bee Pollen

Rich in carbohydrate and protein and containing trace amounts of vitamins and minerals, bee pollen has been used in traditional Chinese medicine to promote general health. It is used today to improve memory and overall performance as well, but at this point there is no concrete scientific evidence to support effectiveness in these areas. Life-threatening reactions may occur after ingestion of bee pollen in individuals who are allergic to pollen or who have asthma. In one published report, a nineteen-year-old male with asthma experienced a serious allergic reaction including severe respiratory distress after taking a commercially processed honeybee-collected pollen supplement. The authors concluded that consumption of processed pollen by individuals with a genetic predisposition to allergies is potentially hazardous and offers little therapeutic benefit.[6]

Bilberry

Historically, bilberry fruit was used to treat diarrhea and scurvy. Today it is taken to treat diarrhea, menstrual cramps, and circulatory problems. Bilberry-plant extract is used to treat diabetes, but this claim has not been verified by scientific studies. It is also believed that bilberry fruit improves night vision, but there is no published scientific data to validate that claim either. However, edible berries such as bilberry, blueberry, cranberry, elderberry, raspberry, and strawberry are potential sources of natural anthocyanin antioxidants, which demonstrate a wide range of health benefits including disease prevention.[7] Consumption of bilberry fruit is safe, but prolonged consumption of bilberry-leaf extract may cause toxicity.

Black Cohosh

Black cohosh is indicated for relieving symptoms of menopause such as night sweats, hot flashes, and vaginal dryness. It is also indicated for inducing labor. This herb is discussed in more detail in Chapter 11.

Burdock

Burdock has been used traditionally to treat arthritis and diabetes. It is also believed to have an anticancer effect and may be effective in lowering blood sugar.

Preliminary studies have indicated that in an animal model, burdock may lower blood sugar. It is an active ingredient of the popular cancer remedy Essiac, and preliminary research indicates that it may be effective in treating various cancers, although data from a large clinical trial is lacking. Although Burdock is considered relatively safe, a 1979 report in the *Journal of the American Medical Association* documents a case of toxicity from consuming a tea prepared from burdock root.

Cat's Claw

Cat's claw is a tropical vine with small thorns at the base of leaves that look like cat's claws, hence the name. This woody vine grows naturally in the rain forests of South America and has been used in South American countries for many centuries to treat various diseases. It is indicated for boosting the immune system, treating viral infections such as herpes, and preventing pregnancy. It is also promoted for treating cancer and arthritis. Clinical research indicates that cat's claw is a potent antioxidant and may inhibit TNF-alpha (tumor necrosis factor, a cytokine produced by red blood cells that plays an important role in inflammation) and prostaglandin synthesis, thus producing beneficial effects in treating osteoarthritis by preventing inflammation.[8] A few side effects such as headache, dizziness, and vomiting have been reported from the use of cat's claw in recommended dosage. Women who are pregnant or trying to get pregnant should avoid cat's claw because it has been traditionally used for preventing pregnancy and inducing abortion.

Capsicum

Capsaicin, which is found in several peppers belonging to the genus *Capsicum*, is believed to have anti-inflammatory properties and may provide relief in ulcers. It is also used for temporary relief of peripheral neuropathies like shingles and minor aches and joint pains. Capsicum extract should be used for short-term pain relief only (one to two days), with a lag period of one to two weeks before the next dose. Severe eye irritation may occur if capsicum extract gets into the eye. Short-term use of capsicum extract is considered safe, and it is on the GRAS list.

Cascara Sagrada

The cured bark of cascara sagrada (*Rhamnus purshiana*), a tree found in British Columbia and the northwestern United States, is a laxative that is available over-the-counter. Cascara tea is also available but has a bitter taste. However, fresh bark should not be consumed as a tea because it contains anthrones, which may cause severe vomiting and abdominal cramps. These compounds can be heat-deactivated or allowed to decompose in storage. Cascara is a safe and effective laxative and is also on the GRAS list.

Chamomile

Chamomile, either Roman or German, is a daisylike, apple-scented flower that has been used in folk medicine for thousands of years. Chamomile essential oil is used for a variety of purposes, including wound healing. As an herbal supplement, chamomile is used to treat anxiety, sleeplessness, upset stomach, and diarrhea. The flowering tops of chamomile plants are used to prepare tea and extracts. Apigenin, found in chamomile, binds with the same receptors as benzodiazepine drugs (used in treating anxiety and insomnia) in mice, and in an animal model it demonstrated sedative and anxiety-relieving effects.[9] Chamomile is safe, but there is some—albeit rare—documentation of allergic reactions, especially in people who are allergic to the daisy family of plants or who suffer from ragweed allergy.[10] Chamomile is in the GRAS list.

Chasteberry

Chasteberry has been used by women for thousands of years to ease menstrual problems and to stimulate production of breast milk. It is indicated today for relief from symptoms of menopause and premenstrual syndrome. Please see Chapter 11 for a detailed discussion.

Cranberry

Cranberry is primarily used to prevent urinary tract infections and is believed to have antiviral, antibacterial, and antioxidant properties. Cranberry is discussed in more detail in Chapter 11.

Damiana

Damiana is a small shrub found in Mexico and Central America. Traditionally it has been used in the form of tea or liquor to increase sexual desire (aphrodisiac). Scientific research indicates that it may contain phytoestrogens (estrogens of plant origin). Essential oil produced from these plants has several medicinal uses, including use as an anti-inflammatory. Damiana is on the GRAS list.

Dandelion

Historically, dandelion has been used to treat liver disease, kidney disease, digestive problems, spleen problems, and as a blood purifier. It is used today as a tonic for the heart and kidneys, to treat minor digestive problems, and as a diuretic. Aqueous extract of dandelion root or herb can produce diuretic effects in rats. The leaves are a rich source of potassium, and loss of potassium as a side effect of diuretic therapy is not observed with dandelion. Scientific research supports the efficacy of dandelion in treating mild digestive disease, as well as its antioxidant, anticancer, and anti-inflammatory effects. These diverse benefits are due to the active polyphenolic compounds and sesquiterpenes in dandelion extract.[11] Extensive clinical data using human trials for dandelion is lacking, but evidence considers dandelion as a generally safe herbal supplement, and it is on the GRAS list.

Dong Quai

Prepared from a Chinese medicinal plant, Dong Quai is an effective remedy for treating menopausal symptoms and other problems associated with women's health. Dong Quai is discussed in detail in Chapter 11.

Echinacea

Echinacea is one of the most commonly sold herbs in the United States, and it has beneficial effects as an immunomodulatory agent. Echinacea can prevent or reduce symptoms of cold and flu and is relatively safe. Echinacea and other immunomodulatory herbs are discussed in Chapter 4.

Evening-Primrose Oil

The oil of evening primrose, a flowering plant native to North America, is indicated for treating eczema, inflammation, and symptoms of rheumatoid arthritis, as well as for relieving premenstrual and menopausal symptoms. The oil is usually put into capsule form for dietary supplementation. Evening-primrose oil has antioxidant properties. Please see Chapter 3 for more discussion on evening-primrose oil.

Fenugreek

Fenugreek seed is used as a cooking spice in many countries, and in many ancient cultures, paste made from fenugreek seeds had a variety of medicinal uses including aiding in childbirth and stimulating lactation. The ancient Chinese used fenugreek as an overall health tonic, and fenugreek is an important component of Indian Ayurvedic medicine. Fenugreek paste is often applied topically to treat many skin problems. As a dietary supplement, fenugreek is indicated for reducing blood sugar and cholesterol, increasing appetite, and treating digestive problems.

Preliminary animal and human trials indicate that fenugreek seed can lower blood sugar and can have beneficial effects on a lipid profile.[12] Abdel-Barry et al. used twenty normal male volunteers between the ages of twenty and thirty to demonstrate that aqueous extract of fenugreek leaves was effective in reducing blood sugar.[13] Patients with diabetes are at an increased risk for cardiovascular disease. A clinical trial has indicated that taking fenugreek-seed powder (25 gm oral dose per day) for twenty-one days reduced cholesterol in five diabetic patients.[14]

Fenugreek is a safe dietary supplement and is on the GRAS list. There are reports of dizziness and diarrhea from using fenugreek, but there is no report of serious adverse effects. Fenugreek may cause abnormally low glucose in diabetic patients taking medicines, so if you are a diabetic, talk to your doctor before using this supplement. Fenugreek may cause bleeding in patients taking warfarin (Coumadin) and, if used with diuretic therapy (water pills), may cause loss of potassium. Animal studies indicate that fenugreek has uterine stimulation properties, and pregnant women should avoid it.

Fennel

Fennel is eaten cooked and raw and is used as a supplement. Traditionally, it has been used for treating upset stomach. Fennel is safe and is on the GRAS list, but there are reports of allergic reactions. People who have seizures and pregnant women should not use fennel. If you are taking the antibiotic ciprofloxacin, you should not take fennel because a study using a rat model showed significant reduction in blood ciprofloxacin levels due to reduced absorption as a result of fennel ingestion.

Feverfew

Feverfew (*Tanacetum parthenium*) is a short perennial bush that grows in fields and along roadsides. Its most common use is for the prevention of migraine headache, but it is also used to relieve arthritis pain, fever, menstrual problems, asthma, and dermatitis. Feverfew is available as fresh leaf, dried powdered leaf, capsules and tablets, fluid extract, and oral drops. The active components of feverfew are parthenolide and other sesquiterpene lactones. During a migraine episode, serotonin is released from platelets, so serotonin antagonists and migraine headache can be treated by inhibiting serotonin release. Research has indicated that using the parthenolide and sesquiterpene lactones present in feverfew can inhibit serotonin release by platelets.[15] E.S. Johnson evaluated the efficacy of feverfew in seventeen patients with at least a two-year history of migraine. The patients took either 50 mg of feverfew or placebo. Patients in the placebo group had migraine more often than patients receiving feverfew.[16] Murphy et al. conducted a randomized double-blind study of feverfew for the prevention of migraine in sixty patients who had suffered migraines for at least two years. All migraine-related medicines were stopped before the study. The patients received one feverfew capsule (70–114 mg) or a placebo four times daily for four months. The number of migraine attacks was significantly lowered in patients taking feverfew.[17] Other natural supplements such as riboflavin, butterbur, and coenzyme Q10 may also be effective in preventing migraine headaches.[18] Although feverfew has an anti-inflammatory effect, clinical trials do not indicate any significant benefit in patients with rheumatoid arthritis.

Feverfew is a relatively safe dietary supplement. Adverse effects associated with its use include dizziness, heartburn, indigestion, bloating, and mouth ulceration. Discontinuation of feverfew may produce muscle and joint stiffness, rebound of migraine symptoms, anxiety, and poor sleep patterns. Feverfew should be avoided during pregnancy. Feverfew also interacts with anticoagulants such as warfarin and with aspirin. Aspirin and nonsteroidal anti-inflammatory drugs (NSAIDS) also have the potential to interact with herbal supplements (bilberry, Dong Quai, garlic, ginger, ginkgo, ginseng, meadowsweet, and willow) that have antiplatelet activities. Aspirin can also interact with chamomile, fenugreek, horse chestnut, and red clover.[19]

Fish Oil

Fish oil is a rich source of omega-3-fatty acids and has many health benefits. It is also relatively safe. Please see Chapter 3 for a more extensive discussion on fish oil.

Flaxseed

Flaxseed (linseed) is most commonly used as a laxative. It is also used to lower high cholesterol and to treat hot flashes, breast pain, and arthritis. Flaxseed contains soluble fiber like that found in oat bran and is a very effective laxative agent. However, due to its high fiber content, it should be taken with plenty of water. Flaxseed contains alpha-linolenic acid, which offers many health benefits. Flaxseed may also have antioxidant and anticancer properties. In one clinical trial involving postmenopausal women not on hormone therapy, flaxseed oil reduced blood total cholesterol and triglyceride levels but had no effect on the markers of bone metabolism (i.e., it did not prevent bone loss).[20]

Flaxseed is a safe and effective dietary supplement. However, it should not be taken with oral medication because its fiber may bind with other drugs, thus preventing a drug from being absorbed from the stomach and entering into the blood circulation. This lowers the effectiveness of the drug, because the blood level of the drug ends up being lower than desired.

Garlic

Garlic is promoted as effective in lowering cholesterol and blood pressure, thus preventing heart attack and stroke. It is also indicated for preventing cancer. Garlic contains various sulfurous compounds, which are derived from allicin. Allicin is formed by the action of an enzyme when garlic is chopped and is responsible for the characteristic odor of garlic. It is mostly destroyed during cooking.

Garlic's historical and worldwide medicinal uses have made it one of the most extensively studied herbal supplements. Clinical trials to determine the lipid-lowering effects of garlic have produced mixed results. Although some studies have not found any statistically significant effects of garlic in lowering serum cholesterol and triglycerides, other studies have shown it to be beneficial. Three clinical trials found 6.1 percent to 11.5 percent reductions in cholesterol in garlic-treated patients, and the reductions were mainly due to reductions in LDL (low-density lipoprotein) or "bad" cholesterol. Triglyceride levels were also decreased after garlic treatment.[21]

Garlic supplement lowered the blood pressure of subjects in some clinical trials, and although not adequately proven, it may reduce the risk of cardiovascular disease.

Garlic is a safe and cheap supplement, and there are only isolated reports of allergic and minor adverse reactions. Garlic is also on the GRAS list. Topically applied garlic may produce allergic reactions in some individuals. Garlic increases the anticoagulant effect of warfarin, and patients on warfarin therapy should not take garlic supplement. However, these patients can use garlic in cooking. The usual dose of garlic supplement is 300 mg two or three times a day. When garlic is cooked, some of its active components, such as allicin, are destroyed. Therefore, garlic supplements contain more concentrations of these active ingredients than cooked garlic. As a result, taking garlic supplements is more effective in lowering cholesterol and obtaining the other beneficial effects of garlic than consuming garlic cooked with other foods.

Chopped-garlic-and-oil mixes left at room temperature can result in fatal botulism (food poisoning), according to the FDA. *Clostridium botulinum* bacteria are dispersed throughout the environment but are not dangerous in the presence of oxygen. The spores produce a deadly toxin in anaerobic (no oxygen), low-acid conditions, causing botulism. The garlic in oil produces that environment. In February 1989, three cases of botulism were reported in persons consuming chopped garlic in oil, which was used as a spread for bread. Testing of leftover garlic in oil showed high concentrations of organism and toxin, and the garlic-in-oil mixture had low acidity (pH 5.7). To avoid food poisoning, it is important to always refrigerate chopped garlic in oil.[22]

> *Garlic has many medicinal benefits and has been widely studied. However, never leave a chopped-garlic-in-oil mix at room temperature; always refrigerate it to avoid food poisoning.*

Ginger

Ginger, like garlic, is a popular culinary and medicinal herb. The ancient Chinese used it as a flavoring agent and in treating nausea. Ginger's characteristic odor and flavor is due to its volatile essential oil. In the United States, ginger is promoted to relieve and prevent nausea caused by motion sickness, morning sickness, and other problems. Ginger is commercially available as the dried powdered root, capsules, tea, oral solution, and as a spice. Some large grocers sell raw ginger root in the produce section. Phillips et al., using 120 patients, studied the efficacy of ginger in preventing postoperative nausea and vomiting. The subjects were given 1 g of ginger, a placebo (no drug), or 100 mg of metoclopramide, an antiemetic medication. The authors concluded that ginger was as effective as metoclopramide in preventing postoperative nausea and vomiting.[23] Clinical research also indicates that ginger is more effective in preventing motion sickness than dimenhydrinate (brand names Dramamine, Gravol, etc.), an over-the-counter medication.

Like garlic, ginger is a safe herbal supplement with no reported serious adverse reactions, and it is on the GRAS list. Mild stomach upset may result in some individuals from ginger supplement.

Ginkgo Biloba

The fruits and seeds of the ginkgo tree have been used in China since ancient times, and the ginkgo tree was brought from China to Europe. Ginkgo biloba is prepared from dried leaves of the tree by organic extraction (acetone/water). After the solvent is removed, the extract is dried and standardized. Most commercial-dosage forms contain 40 mg of this extract. Ginkgo biloba is sold as a dietary supplement for improving blood flow in the brain and extremities, sharpening memory, and to treat vertigo. Ginkgo is one of the best-selling herbs in the United States, and most people take it to prevent age-related dementia and Alzheimer's disease.

The dilemma for researchers is that reports on the benefits of ginkgo are contradictory. Although older studies showed beneficial effects of ginkgo in improving memory and treating dementia due to Alzheimer's disease, a recently published clinical trial showed no such beneficial effects. Wettstein reported that the second-generation cholinesterase inhibitors (metrifonate, donepezil, and rivastigmine, and) and ginkgo extract are equally effective in the treatment of mild to moderate Alzheimer's dementia.[24] In non-Alzheimer's patients, ginkgo can improve memory. In eighteen elderly people who had slight age-related memory loss, ginkgo improved the recall process.[25] However, a recently published clinical trial funded by the National Center for Complementary and Alternative Medicine and conducted between 2000 and 2008 in five academic medical centers involving more than three thousand volunteers aged seventy-five and above did not show any beneficial effects of ginkgo in lowering the overall incidence of dementia and Alzheimer's disease. In this study, volunteers took 120 mg of ginkgo twice a day and were monitored for an average of six years.[26]

One commonly reported adverse effect of ginkgo is bleeding. Spontaneous intracerebral hemorrhage occurred in a seventy-two-year-old woman who was taking 50 mg of ginkgo three times a day for six months.[27] Another report described a seventy-year-old man who presented with bleeding from the iris into the anterior chamber of the eye one week after beginning a self-prescribed regimen consisting of ginkgo-biloba concentrated extract in a dosage of 40 mg twice a day. His medical history included coronary artery bypass surgery performed three years earlier. His only medication was 325 mg of aspirin daily. After the spontaneous-bleeding episode, he continued aspirin but discontinued ginkgo. Over a three-month follow-up period he had no further bleeding episodes. Interaction between ginkgo and aspirin was considered the cause of his eye hemorrhage.[28] Therefore, concurrent use of ginkgo and aspirin as well as other NSAIDS may cause bleeding because ginkgolide B, present in ginkgo extract, is a potent inhibitor of platelet-activating factors. Ginkgo should also be avoided by patients receiving anticoagulant therapy with warfarin because ginkgo increases the action of warfarin and may cause bleeding.

Ginseng

Ginseng is a widely used herbal product in China, other Asian countries, and also in the United States, where it is one of the most common herbal supplements taken by the general population. For thousands of years, people in China have used ginseng as a tonic and also in emergency medicine to rescue dying patients. *Ginseng* means "essence of man" in Chinese. Although the name is used loosely to define many different plants, Asian ginseng, the most common form sold in the United States, is prepared from the root of *Panax ginseng*, which grows naturally in Manchuria. American ginseng is prepared from *Panax quinquefolius*, a related species, while what is called Siberian ginseng is prepared from the root of *Eleutherococcus senticosus*. In the strictest sense, Siberian ginseng is not really a ginseng because it has woody roots instead of the fleshy roots characteristic of true ginseng species. Moreover, the active components of *Eleutheroccus senticosus* differ from those found in true ginseng preparations. Labeling this plant a species of ginseng is believed to have been a marketing ploy. The common preparation of ginseng is from the ginseng root. In the American market, ginseng is sold as liquid extract, tablets, or capsules. Dried ginseng root and ginseng tea are available in health-food stores.

Ginseng is promoted as a tonic capable of invigorating the user physically, mentally, and sexually. Ginseng also has a calming effect. Asian ginseng contains saponins known as ginsenosides; Siberian ginseng does not. Saponins are a class of chemical compounds found primarily in plant species. These compounds form soaplike foam when shaken in water, hence the name saponins. Because of the subjective nature of feeling energy or calmness, it is hard to conduct clinical trials to determine the efficacy of ginseng. One trial involving college students who took 100 mg of ginseng twice daily for twelve weeks showed those who took ginseng performed mathematical calculations at a higher speed than the group that did not. Another study, involving 625 volunteers, concluded that ginseng improved the quality of life among its users.[29] Asian ginseng also has a mild blood-sugar-lowering effect (see Chapter 12). Ginseng may also have an antioxidant effect.

Asian ginseng is a fairly safe supplement. One fatality from the use of ginseng was attributed to contamination of the ginseng product with ephedra.[30] In 1979 the term "ginseng abuse syndrome" was coined as a result of a study of 133 people who took ginseng for one month. Most subjects experienced central nervous system stimulation, but at a higher dose, some experienced confusion and depression. Fourteen patients experienced ginseng abuse syndrome, which is characterized by symptoms of hypertension, nervousness, sleeplessness, skin eruption, and morning diarrhea.[31] Nevertheless, ginseng is considered a generally safe herb for human consumption. Ginseng should be avoided during pregnancy and also by people on anticoagulation therapy with warfarin, since it can reduce that medication's efficacy. Due to ginseng's blood-sugar-lowering effect, people with diabetes taking medication for blood-sugar control should consult their physicians before taking ginseng.

Goldenseal

Goldenseal is indicated for boosting the immune system and for treating colds and respiratory-tract infections. It is also used in wound healing and is often combined with echinacea. This herb is discussed in detail in Chapter 4.

Grape-Seed Extract

Grape-seed extract is indicated for reducing the risk of plaque formation in arteries (atherosclerosis), treating complications related to diabetes, lowering cholesterol, preventing cancer, and healing wounds. Bagchi et al. reported superior antioxidant effects of grape-seed extract (IH636 grape seed proanthocyanidin extract) compared with known antioxidants including vitamin C, vitamin E, and beta-carotene. Moreover, both animal and human studies indicate that grape seed has cardioprotective effects. Grape-seed extract also improved cardiac functions and may also prevent atherosclerosis. The authors concluded that grape-seed extract may be a potential therapeutic tool in promoting cardiovascular health via a number of novel mechanisms.[32] Grape-seed extract is a relatively safe and effective supplement. Clinical trials in which subjects took grape-seed extract up to eight weeks showed no serious safety concerns.

Green Tea

Green teas, including many Chinese and Japanese teas, are consumed as an extract or after brewing. Green-tea extract is intended for lowering cholesterol, improving mental focus, reducing weight, protecting skin from sun damage, and as an antioxidant and anticancer agent. Scientific research has clearly established the antioxidant effect of green tea. Fujiki concluded that 2.5 g of green-tea extract or ten Japanese cups (the small cups used to serve tea in Chinese and Japanese restaurants) of green tea every day may be useful in preventing cancer in a Japanese population.[33] Tea consumption has also been associated with decreased risk of cardiovascular disease. In one clinical trial using theaflavin-enriched green-tea extract on 240 volunteers, the authors demonstrated that it was capable of reducing "bad" cholesterol (LDL or low-density lipoprotein cholesterol) in the blood.[34] Although clinical trials studying the effect of green tea in weight reduction showed mixed results, in one recently published trial, the authors concluded that green tea can reduce body weight in obese Thai subjects by increasing energy expenditure and fat burning.[35]

Green tea and green-tea extract are safe when consumed in moderation, but there are a few reports of acute liver failure due to consumption of green-tea extract. However, the adverse effects of the extract, including liver toxicity, are more likely to occur if the extract is consumed on an empty stomach. If taken on a full stomach or with food, the chances of adverse effects are reduced. Green tea also contains caffeine, and drinking too much green tea may cause insomnia, frequent urination, upset stomach, and diarrhea. Green tea also contains vitamin K, which may reduce the efficacy of the anticoagulant drug warfarin. If you are taking warfarin, please consult your physician before you start taking green-tea extract.

Hawthorn

Hawthorn fruit has historically been used to treat heart disease, especially in European countries. Today, extracts of hawthorn leaves and flowers are indicated for treating heart failure and coronary artery disease. Both liquid extract and dried extract in capsule form are available commercially. Clinical studies have indicated that there is a significant benefit in symptom control and physiological outcome from hawthorn extract as an adjunct treatment for chronic heart failure.[36] Hawthorn is safe for most adults when used for a short period, and side effects are minimal.

Horse Chestnut

For centuries, the seeds, leaves, bark, and flowers of the horse chestnut tree have been used to improve poor blood circulation (chronic venous insufficiency) in order to treat varicose veins, ankle swelling, nighttime leg cramps, and hemorrhoids. Homemade horse-chestnut preparations should not be used because raw seeds contain esculin, a poison. Properly processed horse-chestnut preparation does not contain this poison. Clinical trials have clearly indicated that horse-chestnut seed extract is effective in treating chronic venous insufficiency.[37] Aescin, the active component of horse-chestnut-seed extract, is responsible for its pharmacological action.[38] Horse-chestnut-seed extract is a safe and effective herbal supplement. Short-term use of horse-chestnut-seed extract may help in relieving pain, ankle and leg swelling (edema), and leg cramps. The long-term safety of horse chestnut has not been reported, so this herbal supplement should not be used for a long period of time.

Lavender

Oil from the lavender plant is an essential oil used mainly in aromatherapy and also by the perfume industry. Aromatherapy using lavender essential oil has many health benefits, which are discussed in detail in Chapter 3. Lavender is on the GRAS list.

Licorice

Licorice root has been used in Indian Ayurvedic medicine, Asian medicine, and in European countries for many centuries. Licorice extract has a sweet taste and is often used as a flavoring agent to mask the bitter taste of preparations and in making candy. It is also used as an expectorant. Licorice root has been used as a dietary supplement for treating stomach ulcers, bronchitis, and sore throat. It is also indicated for treating viral illness such as hepatitis C. Licorice is available as a liquid root extract or as a dried powder in capsule form. The main component of licorice extract is glycyrrhizic acid, although it contains a variety of other active compounds, such as triterpene saponins and flavonoids, as well.

Clinical studies have reported beneficial effects of both licorice and glycyrrhizin consumption, including antiulcer, antiviral, and protection of the liver from injury. If consumed for a long time or in high amounts, licorice extract may inhibit the activity of the enzyme that inactivates cortisol. This effect is reversed when licorice is discontinued. Otherwise, licorice is a safe and effective supplement.[39] In addition, licorice-root extract has cardioprotective, anticancer, and steroidlike anti-inflammatory properties. It is effective in protecting the liver from hepatitis A– and hepatitis B–induced damage; it can stop the replication of the hepatitis C virus and may eventually kill the virus.[40] Use of licorice-root extract for four to six weeks is safe and usually does not produce any serious adverse effects.

Licorice is on the GRAS list. However, glycyrrhizin consumption may increase blood pressure. People suffering from high blood pressure are advised not to take any licorice supplement without consulting their physician. If you are taking a water pill (diuretic), you should not take a licorice supplement without approval from your physician, as it may increase potassium loss, resulting in serious symptoms.

Lutein

Lutein is a carotenoid found in green leafy vegetables such as spinach and also in fruits, vegetables, and egg yolk. Lutein is found in the human retina, and people who consume high amounts of vegetables each day are less likely to have certain eye diseases such as macular degeneration. Lutein also protects the eye against the formation of cataracts and has antioxidant properties. In one study, the authors concluded that higher intake of lutein through lutein-enriched fruits and vegetables enabled patients with age-related cataracts to have better visual function. Lutein is a safe and effective supplement with no known adverse effects reported. A lutein supplement of 10 mg per day has been shown to be safe for a one-year period.[41]

Lycopene

Lycopene, a red pigment found mostly in tomatoes but also in strawberries and watermelon, is an antioxidant and has potential protective effects against cancer, especially prostate cancer. Studies have shown that consumption of tomatoes and tomato products is associated with low risk of developing prostate cancer. Lycopene supplementation is safe, and no adverse effect has been identified.[42]

Milk Thistle

For more than two thousand years, seeds of milk thistle have been used to treat liver disease. In the United States, milk thistle is mainly used to treat viral infection and cirrhosis of the liver. An active component of milk thistle, silymarin, protects the liver from a variety of liver toxins in animal models.[43] Clinical trials to evaluate the efficacy of milk thistle in treating liver cirrhosis reported mixed results. In one trial, the authors found that milk thistle had beneficial effects for those patients who had mild alcoholic liver cirrhosis. In another trial, the blood tests for liver damage showed improvement in cirrhosis patients who took milk-thistle supplements. However, other studies reported no beneficial effect in treating liver cirrhosis with milk-thistle supplements. Milk thistle is beneficial as a supportive therapy in treating mushroom (*Amanita phalloides*) poisoning.[44] Clinical trials also indicate that milk thistle may have anticancer and antidiabetic effects and may also lower serum cholesterol. Milk-thistle extracts are known to be safe and well tolerated, and adverse reactions are usually minimal.[45]

Noni

Noni is an evergreen shrub that grows throughout tropical regions of the South Pacific islands. Traditionally, people used the leaves and fruits of noni to make juice, which they drank as a health tonic. Today, people also drink noni juice to treat diabetes and cardiovascular disease. Noni extract is applied topically for relief from joint pain. Clinical studies indicate that noni juice may help in combating fatigue. In addition, it may have antiviral, antifungal, analgesic, and anti-inflammatory effects. Noni juice is effective in boosting the immune system and may also protect against cancer.[46] Noni juice is high in potassium and should not be consumed by people on potassium-restricted diets.

The safety of noni juice has not been evaluated completely. There are two cases of liver damage resulting from its consumption. A twenty-nine-year-old man with previous toxic hepatitis due to acetaminophen use developed acute hepatic failure after consumption of 1.5 L of noni juice over three weeks. The patient underwent a liver transplant. A sixty-two-year-old woman with no previous report of liver injury developed self-limiting acute hepatitis following the consumption of 2 L of noni juice over a period of three months.[47] If you have any liver problems or hepatitis, you should not take noni juice.

Osha

Osha is an herbal supplement indicated for boosting the immune system and for preventing cold and flu. It is also used in relieving symptoms of a cold. See Chapter 4 for a more detailed discussion of osha.

Peppermint Oil

Peppermint oil has been used for treating a variety of symptoms including nausea, indigestion, cold, headache, and irritable bowel syndrome. Peppermint essential oil has many beneficial effects. See Chapter 3 for a more in-depth discussion on the health benefits of peppermint oil. Peppermint oil is on the GRAS list.

Red Clover

The flowering tops of the red-clover plant are used to prepare extracts that are indicated for relieving menopausal symptoms, breast pain, high cholesterol, osteoporosis, and symptoms of prostate enlargement. Red clover has also been used in treating respiratory problems such as cough, asthma, and bronchitis. Red clover is discussed in more detail in Chapter 11. It is on the GRAS list.

Saw Palmetto

Saw palmetto is a dwarf palm tree that grows in the southern United States. Native Americans used saw palmetto to treat genitourinary conditions. In the early twentieth century it was used in conventional medicine as a mild diuretic and as a treatment for benign prostatic hypertrophy (BPH). Today, this herbal supplement is mostly taken to treat an enlarged prostate. The recommended dose is 1–2 g of dried saw-palmetto fruit or 320 mg of lipophilic extract. Carraro et al. performed a large double-blind study evaluating the efficacy of saw palmetto for the treatment of BPH using 1,098 men with moderate BPH and observed no benefit.[48] However, in another clinical trial using 44 men, the authors observed a slight advantage of saw palmetto in treating BPH.[49] Adverse effects appear to be minimal, mostly gastrointestinal upset. Although no interaction between Western drugs and saw palmetto has been reported, the use of saw palmetto with other hormonal therapy may have additive effects. Therefore, if you are receiving any hormonal therapy, please get your physician's approval before taking saw palmetto. Saw palmetto does not affect the laboratory test for prostate cancer (PSA, prostate-specific antigen).

Senna

Senna is used mainly as a laxative. In the United States it is available as leaf extract, fruit extract, or powder. When used in recommended doses, senna laxative is safe and effective if taken for a short duration (less than seven days). Senna is on the GRAS list of safe botanical supplements. However, abuse of senna may cause problems due to loss of potassium as well as abdominal pain, severe diarrhea, and weight loss. There is a case report of acute liver failure in a fifty-two-year-old woman who ingested very large amounts of senna fruit as an herbal tea. For over three years she ingested 1 liter of herbal tea a day from a bag containing 70 g of dry senna fruit. She developed acute liver failure and renal impairment, requiring admission to the intensive-care unit of the hospital.[50] Although this is the only report indicating an adverse effect when senna is consumed in excess, it is better to stick to the recommended dosage of senna and not to consume too much.

Soy

Soy is available as a dietary supplement in the form of tablets and capsules and may contain soy proteins, isoflavones, or both. Soybeans can be cooked and eaten or can be used to make soy milk, tofu, or other food products. Soy supplementation is indicated for lowering cholesterol, weight loss, and relieving symptoms of menopause such as hot flashes and osteoporosis. It is believed that soy supplementation can also prevent cancer and improve memory. Soy protein is a complete protein because it contains ample amounts of all essential amino acids and several other nutrients. Therefore, it is considered equivalent to animal protein. Soy also contains isoflavones, a group of compounds with many beneficial effects. Several studies using both human and animal models have indicated that consumption of soy protein reduces body weight and fat mass. In obese humans, soy supplement reduces body weight and fat mass in addition to reducing cholesterol and triglycerides.[51] Soy supplement reduces cholesterol via a novel mechanism, activating receptors in the liver that remove "bad" (LDL, or low-density lipoprotein) cholesterol from the blood.[52] Another study indicates that soy consumption reduces the incidence of hot flashes in menopausal women.[53] However, the cancer-prevention capacity of soy supplement has not been demonstrated by rigorous research.

Soy is an effective and safe supplement with only a few reported minor side effects. Some people may experience nausea, bloating, or constipation following the consumption of soy supplement. In rare cases, allergic reaction and rash occur. However, consumption of excess soy may cause several serious adverse effects such as bowel problems, digestive problems, a breaking down of the immune system, and even increased risk of heart disease and cancer. In addition, soy contains several compounds that are similar to female hormones (plant estrogens), and experiments with monkeys indicate that if a male consumes soy on a regular basis, he may experience some nonspecific symptoms.

St. John's Wort

St. John's wort is prepared from a perennial aromatic shrub with bright yellow flowers that bloom from June to September. The flowers are believed to be brightest and most abundant on or near June 24, the day traditionally believed to be the birthday of John the Baptist. Therefore, the name St. John's wort became popular for this plant. The flowering tops, leaves, or stems are used to make extracts or dried powder for prepared capsules. St. John's wort is one of the best-selling herbal supplements in the United States and is mostly used for treating depression, anxiety, and sleep disorders. Many chemicals have been isolated from St. John's wort, with hypericin and hyperforin mainly responsible for the anti-depressant effects. Most commercially available St.-John's-wort preparations are standardized to contain 0.3 percent hypericin. Linde et al. analyzed data from twenty-three clinical trials involving St. John's wort (1,757 outpatients) and concluded that it is effective in treating mild to moderate depression. In addition, based on data from eight of these studies, it was suggested that St. John's wort has equivalent efficacy to low-dose treatment with antidepressant medications (amitriptyline or imipramine). Interestingly, St. John's wort has fewer side effects than these medications.[54] A recent study also indicated that St.-John's-wort extract has a meaningful beneficial effect during acute treatment of patients suffering from mild depression and leads to a substantial increase in the probability of remission.[55] However, St. John's wort is not effective in treating major depression and is not considered a proven therapy for depression. If you are taking St. John's wort for depression and your depression persists, please see a physician, as depression may cause severe health problems if untreated by a professional.

St. John's wort is fairly safe and is on the GRAS list, but it may induce photosensitivity, especially in fair-skinned persons, following exposure to sunlight or UV light. After taking St. John's wort for four weeks, a thirty-five-year-old woman complained about stinging pain on sun-exposed areas. Her symptoms improved two months after she discontinued the product.[56] There are a few case reports describing episodes of hypomania (irritability, disinhibition, agitation, anger, insomnia, and difficulty concentrating) after using St. John's wort. The major problem with taking this supplement is its reported interactions with many Western drugs. St. John's wort induces liver enzymes, which metabolize many drugs, thus reducing effective blood levels of the drugs. In addition, by other complex mechanisms, St. John's wort reduces blood levels of many drugs that are not primarily metabolized by the liver. Therefore, treatment failure may result. In particular, patients receiving warfarin therapy, transplant recipients, and patients being treated for AIDS may face serious treatment failure if they begin taking St. John's wort. Please see Chapter 9 for a more detailed discussion on drug interactions with St. John's wort.

> *If you are taking any medication on a regular basis for the treatment of a chronic health problem, do not take St. John's wort without approval from your physician.*

Turmeric

Turmeric is an Indian plant that is used as a spice in many Asian countries and is an important component of traditional Chinese and Indian Ayurvedic medicine. Turmeric's fingerlike underground stems (rhizomes) are dried for use as a spice and taken as a powder in capsule form. Liquid extract of turmeric is also commercially available. Turmeric can also be used as a paste for application on the skin. The most active component of turmeric is curcumin. Scientific research has shown that turmeric has antibacterial, antiviral, antifungal, antioxidant, and anticancer activities and thus has a potential against various malignant diseases, arthritis, Alzheimer's disease, and other chronic illnesses.[57] Turmeric is also very effective in preventing rheumatoid arthritis.[58]

Turmeric is a safe and effective herbal supplement and is on the GRAS list. High doses and long-term use may cause indigestion. People with gallbladder disease should avoid using a turmeric supplement.

Valerian

Valerian is a perennial herb that grows in North America, Europe, and western Asia. The crude valerian root, rhizome, or stolon is dried and is used as a powder or as an extract. Valerian is available as a capsule, liquid extract, or tea and is used as a sleeping aid. More than forty compounds have been isolated from valerian root, with valepotriates probably responsible for the sedative effect. Valerenic acid, another component of valerian, may also produce sedative effects. Leathwood conducted a study with 128 volunteers and concluded that valerian significantly improved subjective sleep quality in habitually poor or irregular sleepers.[59] Another more recent study demonstrated that a combination of valerian and hops is an effective sleeping aid. Valerian supports readiness to go to sleep, while hops has a sleep-inducing, melatonin-like effect. The authors concluded that based on their investigation, the efficacy of valerian and hops combined to treat sleep disorder can be explained from a scientific point of view.[60]

Studies have indicated that valerian is generally safe if used for a short-term period (four to six weeks) for the relief of insomnia. The long-term safety of valerian has not been reported. Side effects, including dizziness, upset stomach, headache, and morning sleepiness, are generally mild. Valerian is on the GRAS list.

Other Dietary Supplements

Other than herbal supplements, people also take a variety of dietary supplements that are not directly prepared from medicinal plants. These include various amino acids, chondroitin, coenzyme Q10, glucosamine, melatonin, probiotics, and vitamins and minerals. The efficacy of vitamins and minerals as dietary supplements are discussed in Chapter 6.

Amino-Acid Supplements

Amino-acid supplements are recommended for promoting general well-being and for building muscle and muscle strength. Amino acids are the building block of proteins and are essential for life. We need twenty amino acids, and of these, nine are considered essential (histidine, leucine, isoleucine, methionine, phenylalanine, threonine, tryptophan, and valine) because they cannot be produced by our bodies and must be obtained from our food. Protein-rich foods such as meat, fish, dairy products, eggs, legumes, soy, and nuts can provide our daily requirements. If we eat a balanced diet and are healthy, we do not suffer from amino-acid deficiency and do not require supplements. Contrary to the popular belief that these supplements may increase stamina and endurance, research indicates that branched-chain amino acids do not improve endurance, and the evidence that a glutamine supplement may improve immune function is rather weak. In addition, commercial supplements contain too little arginine to increase growth-hormone levels.[61]

However, occasionally amino-acid supplements are used to treat a deficiency of an individual amino acid, which may occur due to a digestive disorder, critical illness, or genetic factors. Your doctor can order blood tests to determine which supplement is best suited to treat your condition. Amino-acid supplements, if taken in excess, can cause toxicity and may even harm you.

Coenzyme Q10

Coenzyme Q10, a fat-soluble, vitamin-like compound, is naturally produced in our cells, but as we age its concentration is usually reduced. It can be found in supplements as a single ingredient or in combination with other ingredients. These products account for over $200 million in sales in the United States annually. Discovered in 1957, coenzyme Q10 plays a vital role in energy metabolism in cells. It also has antioxidant properties and is indicated for treating a variety of diseases including Parkinson's and other neurological diseases, migraines, cardiovascular disease, and diabetes. Because coenzyme Q10 is sold as a dietary supplement, no claim for its therapeutic benefits can be made according to the 1994 law. In Japan, coenzyme Q10 is approved for treating congestive heart failure. It appears to be most promising for neurodegenerative diseases such as Parkinson's.[62] Clinical studies clearly indicate that coenzyme Q10 is beneficial in treating heart failure and high blood pressure but is less effective in treating ischemic heart disease, a disease characterized by reduced blood supply in the heart due to the formation of atherosclerotic plaques in the arteries.[63] Its efficacy in treating diabetes is controversial, as studies have produced conflicting results. Coenzyme Q10 is a safe dietary supplement if taken in recommended dosages, and reports of adverse effects are rare. However, it can interact with many drugs such as the anticoagulant warfarin, cholesterol-lowering drugs, diabetic medicines, and antidepressants.

> **If you are taking any medications for a chronic illness, do not take coenzyme Q10 without your doctor's approval.**

Creatine

Athletes use creatine (such as creatine monohydrate) supplements to improve performance. (Creatine is not a steroid; it is produced by the body, then broken down to creatinine, which is excreted in urine and is structurally very different from a steroid.) Creatine is synthesized in our bodies from amino acids mostly by the kidney, liver, and pancreas, and it is found predominately in muscle (approximately 40 percent in free form and 60 percent as creatine phosphate). Creatine is involved in energy metabolism; its breakdown product, creatinine, is excreted by the kidneys and is used as a marker to evaluate renal function. A creatine supplement of 20 g per day for three days has resulted in creatinine concentrations in some subjects but not in all, indicating that there are responders and nonresponders. Creatine is usually low in vegetarians, and they respond well to creatine supplement. Although some studies have indicated improved performance in subjects taking creatine, other studies failed to document such effects. Creatine supplement does not improve endurance and incremental-type exercise and may even be detrimental.[64] It also offers little benefit in preventing muscle damage and soreness but may improve performance in activities such as jumping, sprinting, and cycling. Creatine supplement is safe if taken short-term, but its long-term safety is not known.

DHEA

DHEA (dehydroepiandrosterone) is a hormone secreted by the adrenal gland; its levels decrease with age. DHEA (often sold as DHEA sulfate) is used as a dietary supplement, but clinical trials evaluating its efficacy in treating various diseases have shown inconsistent results and its use is currently very controversial. Pharmacological studies have suggested that dosages of 30–50 mg may increase blood testosterone levels in women, resulting in increased libido; however, no such effect was observed in males. DHEA may be effective in treating patients with adrenal insufficiency, and these patients may experience improved sexual function, increased self-esteem, and decreased fatigue. However, research studying the efficacy of DHEA supplementation in treating patients with lupus, Alzheimer's disease, HIV, male sexual dysfunction, menopausal symptoms, depression, and cardiovascular disease has not produced consistent findings.[65]

Glucosamine and Chondroitin

Glucosamine is either produced synthetically or is derived from the skeletons of marine animals. Clinical trials have indicated that glucosamine is effective in relieving pain resulting from osteoarthritis, especially knee pain, and can slow the progression of the disease.

Chondroitin is prepared from shark or bovine cartilage. In combination with iron, chondroitin is used in treating anemia. Chondroitin alone or in combination with glucosamine is used to treat osteoarthritis, and the two in combination have been shown to be effective in treating joint pain due to osteoarthritis. Adverse effects from glucosamine and chondroitin are rare.[66]

L-Carnitine

L-isomer of carnitine, known as L-carnitine, is a water-soluble amino acid that plays an important role in transporting fatty acids inside cells for breakdown so that cells can obtain energy. L-carnitine is essential for muscular activity, and deficiency produces muscle weakness. We normally get enough L-carnitine from food (meat, poultry, fish, peanut butter, asparagus, avocado, and other fruits and vegetables), and at this point research indicates that unless we have carnitine deficiency, there is no health benefit in taking carnitine supplement. However, studies indicate that L-carnitine supplement may be useful after a heart attack, congestive heart failure, and in treating chronic fatigue syndrome; it may also help improve exercise performance. Treatment with valproic acid, a chemical compound used as an anticonvulsive and as a mood stabilizer, may lower blood carnitine levels, in which case L-carnitine supplementation may be helpful. Carnitine is also an antidote to severe valproic-acid toxicity, especially in children.[67] Carnitine-replacement therapy in dialysis patients, however, is a controversial issue.

Melatonin

Melatonin, a hormone secreted by the pineal gland of the brain, regulates the body's twenty-four–hour clock (circadian rhythm), helping us go to sleep and wake up again. Its production is stimulated by darkness and suppressed by light. It also controls the timing of the release of female reproductive hormones, thus playing a role in regulating menstrual cycles. Melatonin is remarkably effective in preventing or reducing jet lag—especially for adult travelers flying across five or more time zones, particularly in an eastward direction. It may also be helpful for traveling across two to four time zones.[68] Melatonin supplement is a safe and effective strategy to slow the aging process due to its antioxidant effect.[69] It may help to alleviate symptoms of mild depression because people with depression often have low levels of melatonin. Melatonin may also help women control menopausal symptoms for a short period. The cancer-preventive action of melatonin has not been established.

Probiotics

Probiotics, which are "friendly" bacteria, are living microorganisms that have potential health benefits. Most commercially available probiotic combinations contain lactobacillus or bifidobacterium and their various species. Other common probiotics are yeasts. *Lactobacillus acidophilus*, which is found in milk and yogurt, protects humans against "bad" bacteria. It works by leading to the production of lactic acid and hydrogen peroxide when food breaks down, and both lactic acid and hydrogen peroxide can kill bacteria. *Lactobacillus acidophilus* also produces lactase, which breaks down milk sugar (lactose). People with lactose intolerance do not produce this enzyme and may benefit from taking a dietary supplement containing *Lactobacillus acidophilus*. Probiotics reinforce the integrity of the intestinal lining as a barrier to harmful bacteria. In addition, they keep the growth of harmful bacteria and yeast under control, which is why women use acidophilus for yeast infections. Clinical studies have shown that probiotic supplements are an effective way to prevent traveler's diarrhea. Probiotics may also be helpful to patients suffering from ulcerative colitis.[70]

Weight-Loss Products

After the FDA banned the use of herbal weight-loss products containing ephedra, many other supplements appeared on the market. Many of these contain chromium, but clinical trials have not established the efficacy of chromium in weight loss. In addition, the long-term safety of chromium is not known. Numerous weight-loss products contain soluble fibers including guar gum, glucomannan, and psyllium, but clinical studies have not shown any weight-loss benefit to these either. However, dietary fibers have other health benefits such as reducing absorption of lipids from the gut. Similarly, there is no clinical data supporting the efficacy of both hydroxy citric acid and linoleic acid in weight loss. Green tea may be effective in weight loss. Currently, there is no data on the efficacy of guggul and apple cider vinegar in weight loss.[71]

Conclusion

Many herbal supplements have documented benefits and are fairly safe to consume. However, it is always advised that you inform your doctor about your use of herbal supplements so that if you develop any unusual condition, your doctor can determine whether that condition is due to the use of herbal supplements.

CHAPTER 3

Essential Oils and Fish-Oil Supplements: How Effective Are They?

The term "lipid" generally refers to a wide group of biomolecules including fats, oils (liquid fat; both solid and liquid fats and oils are composed of various fatty acids and exist as complex molecules called triglycerides), phospholipids, glycolipids, and various sterols. The most commonly encountered sterol is cholesterol. These molecules are building blocks of the animal kingdom because phospholipids and cholesterol are major components of cell membrane. In addition, fats play a major role in energy storage, oxygen transport, control of inflammation, intercellular communication, blood clotting, and a variety of other complex biochemical processes essential for sustaining life. Vegetable oils and essential oils are major sources of fatty acids, including essential fatty acids.

Essential Fatty Acids (Omega-3 and Omega-6 Fatty Acids)

Fatty acids are composed of carbon, hydrogen, and oxygen atoms linked or bonded in different ways. There are two types of fatty acids: saturated and unsaturated, distinguished by differences in the geometry and number of carbon bonds, which also influence their function in the body. The human body can produce all but two of the fatty acids it needs: linoleic acid (LA) and alpha-linolenic acid (ALA). These are found in plant oils and, since they cannot be made in the body and must be obtained from food, they are called essential fatty acids. In the body, essential fatty acids are primarily used to produce hormonelike substances (prostaglandins and thromboxanes) that regulate a wide range of functions, including blood pressure, blood clotting, blood lipid levels, the immune response, and the inflammation response to injury infection. Fatty acids also play an important role in the life and death of cardiac cells because they are essential fuels for the mechanical and electrical activities of the heart.

Oleic acid (the major constituent of olive oil) has only one carbon double bond, while in linoleic acid (present in many vegetable oils) there are two. In fatty acids found in fish oil, five or even six double carbon bonds may be present. When more than one double bond is present in a fatty acid, it is termed a polyunsaturated fatty acid.

There are two series of unsaturated fatty acids (see Figure 3.1). In omega-3 fatty acids, the first double carbon bond is encountered at carbon atom number 3, while in omega-6 fatty acids, the first double bond is encountered at carbon atom number 6. Dietary alpha-linolenic acid is the precursor of omega-3 fatty acids such as eicosapentaenoic acid and docosahexaenoic acid, which are found in abundance in fish, while linolenic acid is the precursor of omega-6 fatty acids. In general, fish oils contain longer-chain omega-3 fatty acids, which help to fulfill the body's requirement of essential fatty acids and may have beneficial properties of their own.

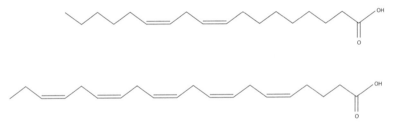

FIGURE 3.1: The chemical structures of an omega-3 and an omega-6 fatty acid

Our body requires both omega-3 and omega-6 fatty acids. While we get plenty of omega-6 fatty acids through our diet (grains, meat, milk, eggs, vegetable oils, etc.), omega-3 fatty acids are less readily found; certain foods, including fish and nuts, provide abundant amounts. Deficiency in omega-3 fatty acids may cause a dry, scaly rash, make the skin prone to infection, and cause poor wound healing. In children, a deficiency in this type of fatty acid may cause poor development. However, in developed countries, essential fatty acid deficiency due to a poor diet is relatively uncommon compared to in poor countries. Some essential oils, such as evening-primrose oil, are rich in omega-3 fatty acids.

Unsaturated fatty acids can be further classified into two categories: cis-fatty acids and trans-fatty acids. These types differ in the way the double bond is arranged in the fatty-acid molecule. Trans-fatty acids are found in animal fat and are also produced by bacterial metabolism. Four percent of milk is comprised of trans-fatty acids. In contrast, cis-fatty acids are found in plants and are present in plant oils used for cooking. Trans-fatty acids, just like saturated fatty acids, can increase "bad" cholesterol (LDL cholesterol) and lower "good" cholesterol (HDL cholesterol), and may also increase the risk of various heart diseases, including heart attack.

Essential Oils

Essential oils prepared from aromatic plants are water-insoluble (hydrophobic) liquids containing various volatile aromatic compounds. The oil is called "essential" because each oil specimen carries the distinct essence (fragrance) of the plant from which it is prepared. Essential oils can come from various parts of a plant including the berries, seeds, bark, wood, rhizomes, leaves, resin, flowers, peel, and roots (see Table 3.1). These oils are generally extracted from a plant by a steam distillation process, by mechanical pressing, or through the use of solvents. Usually, large amounts of plant materials are required to extract a good quantity of essential oil.

TABLE 3.1: Plant Parts Used in Making Essential Oils

PLANT PART	ESSENTIAL OIL
Bark	Cinnamon, sassafras
Berries	Juniper
Flowers	Chamomile, clove, jasmine, lavender, orange, rose
Leaves	Basil, cinnamon, eucalyptus, oregano, peppermint, rosemary, sage, tea tree, thyme, wintergreen
Peel	Grapefruit, lemon, lime, orange
Rhizome (underground stems)	Galangal, ginger
Root	Valerian
Seeds	Almond, cumin, nutmeg
Wood	Cedar, rosewood, sandalwood

The pharmaceutical properties of aromatic plants are attributed to essential oils, which contain many terpene and nonterpene compounds that have various pharmacological activities. Many essential oils have antibacterial, antifungal, antiviral, and antioxidant properties. In addition, some essential oils may play a role in preventing heart diseases. Massage and aromatherapy using essential oils also offer health benefits.[1]

Essential oils have been used in medicine from prehistoric times, and they played an important part in ancient Ayurvedic medicinal practice in India. When the Buddha (who was born five hundred years before Christ) was suffering from severe headache, Jivaka, the most eminent physician in the kingdom of Emperor Ashok, cured him using aromatherapy. Aromatherapy is currently used worldwide for the management of chronic pain, depression, anxiety, insomnia, some cognitive disorders, and stress-related disorders.[2]

Essential oils can be used in a variety of ways, including diffusion into the air for their distinct scent, direct or indirect inhalation, as an additive to laundry detergent or to bathwater, and in aromatherapy and massage. They can be used to treat skin rash and heal wounds as well as in dietary supplements (such as Evening-primrose oil). It should be noted that unlike vegetable oils, essential oils have active components such as linalool, carvacrol, thymol, camphor, and eugenol and may be toxic if ingested. They should be kept out of reach of children—in the Western world, essential oils are the fourth-most common agent in childhood poisoning.[3] Poisoning from the consumption of oil of wintergreen is usually fatal in children because it contains high amounts methyl salicylate, which is structurally related to aspirin (acetylsalicylate). Although acetylsalicylate can be taken orally, methyl salicylate is a known poison and should not be ingested. Five mL of oil of wintergreen is equivalent to 21.7 adult aspirin tablets (325 mg),[4] and its ingestion can cause serious toxicity even in adults.

> *The ingestion of as little as 4 ml of oil of wintergreen can be fatal to a child.*

CASE STUDY

The mother of a fifteen-month-old boy had a toothache and was using clove oil to relieve it. Early one morning the child was playing alone near the bottle while his mother was in the bathroom, and he accidentally ingested clove oil. He got very sick and was rushed to the emergency room. Later he developed liver failure, as evidenced by his blood tests. Even forty-eight hours after ingestion of clove oil, he was still lethargic. Clove oil contains eugenol, a known liver toxin. Fortunately, the boy's condition improved slowly over a period of eight days as he was treated with N-acetylcysteine.[5]

A four-year-old boy ingested a small quantity of tea-tree oil, and within thirty minutes he developed irregular breathing and shortly afterward became unresponsive. Paramedics were called and he was intubated for artificial respiration. After proper medical attention, his neurological condition improved gradually over next the ten hours, and he recovered.[6]

In addition to keeping essential oils out of reach of children, you should store them in tightly capped bottles in a cold location away from light. People with allergies or sensitive skin should use extreme caution when applying essential oils, and it is always best to consult with a qualified herbalist or a health-care provider before using one. It is also wise not to apply essential oil on the skin of small babies, as their skin is much too sensitive. Also, since essential oils are not water-soluble, keep carrier oil (e.g., olive, grape seed, almond, jojoba, etc.) handy so that in case an essential oil causes an unwanted skin reaction, it can be diluted with vegetable oil.

Essential oils are very potent, and one or two drops should be enough to produce benefits. Some essential oils can be applied directly onto the skin, while dilution with carrier oil is recommended for others. Similarly, adding two to three drops of essential oil to bath gel or shampoo is enough to produce maximum effect. For inhalation, two drops can be put into your palm or a handkerchief. For massage, mix a few drops of essential oil with massage oil. Although a few essential oils are safe as dietary supplements, be cautious when using essential oils this way because they can be toxic. It is not a good idea to start taking an essential oil as a dietary supplement based on the recommendation of friends or relatives who are neither herbalists nor medically qualified.

> *If you wish to take an essential oil, consult a qualified herbalist or a naturopathic doctor to determine if you are likely to derive any benefit. If you do use essential oil as a dietary supplement, it is wise to do so for only a short period of time, such as less than a week, unless your doctor approves use for a longer period.*

Active components of essential oils are often volatile, and inhalation can produce many benefits. Similarly, applying essential oil topically produces many beneficial effects because small molecules of essential oil can penetrate your skin.

> *Be careful not to get any essential oil into your eyes. If you do, seek medi-*
> *cal help, because essential oils cannot be removed from eyes simply by*
> *washing with water.*

Many essential oils of citrus origin, such as lemon oil,[7] cause photosensitivity because they contain active components such as furocoumarin derivatives, which have phototoxic activities. If you use any of these oils on your skin, avoid exposing it to sunlight or direct UV light (for example, in a tanning salon) for several days. Kaddu et al. described two cases where patients developed phototoxic skin reactions within forty-eight to seventy-two hours after exposure to bergamot aromatherapy oil (an extract from the rind of bergamot orange, which has a refreshing scent) followed by ultraviolet exposure.[8]

> *Lemon, orange, bergamot, tangerine, grapefruit, and other citrus-based*
> *oils may cause skin rash or dark pigmentation on skin that is exposed to*
> *sunlight or UV light up to two to three days after application.*

Commonly Used Essential Oils

An estimated three thousand essential oils are known, and around three hundred are commercially important to the fragrance market. Essential oils such as aniseed, calamus, camphor, cinnamon, clove, eucalyptus, orange, lemongrass, rosemary, and basil are used worldwide for various purposes.[9] Commonly used essential oils are listed in Table 3.2. Scientific research indicates that cinnamon, clove, and rosemary oil have antibacterial properties.[10] Basil oil has anti-inflammatory properties, while lemon and rosemary oils have antioxidant properties.[11] Citronella oil is an antifungal, while lavender oil offers both antifungal and antibacterial benefits. Lavender oil is effective in treating insect bites and burns.[12] However, lavender oil lacks natural protection from autoxidation (oxidation by direct combination with oxygen at ordinary temperatures), a process that causes the oil to produce a class of chemicals called hydroperoxides, which are allergens.[13] In order to avoid allergic reactions from the use of lavender oil in aromatherapy, it is essential to prepare your blend of oil just previous to starting therapy. Lavender oil should be kept tightly capped in a small bottle to avoid exposure to air.

TABLE 3.2: Commonly Used Essential Oils

ESSENTIAL OIL	USE
Aniseed	Expectorant; oil vapor useful in treating cold, flu
Basil	Antibacterial, insecticidal, aromatherapeutic
Bergamot	Aromatherapeutic, perfume
Chamomile (Roman and German)	Calming, aromatherapeutic; vapor helps to relieve headache, migraine
Calamus	Local analgesic, anti-inflammatory, aromatherapeutic
Camphor	Vapor used for relieving respiratory problems; should not be used as an aromatherapeutic because it can be toxic
Cedarwood	Abortifacient, antiseptic, insecticide, perfume, aromatherapeutic
Cinnamon	Antibacterial, antiseptic, flavoring agent
Citronella	Perfume, mosquito repellent
Clove	Dental analgesic, antiseptic
Cypress	Aromatherapeutic; oil vapor helps control cough, cold, bronchitis
Eucalyptus	Antibacterial; vapor therapy useful for control of sneezing, hay fever; used in bath for relief of arthritis pain
Geranium	Mild analgesic, sedative, minor burn remedy
Grapefruit	Antiseptic, disinfectant; protects against cold, flu; massage oil
Hyssop	Cleanser and detoxifier
Jasmine	Soothing and calming; vapor therapy useful for relaxation; helps with depression
Lavender	Aromatherapeutic, antibacterial; helps treat acne and burns
Lemon	Perfume, flavoring agent
Orange	Perfume, flavoring agent
Peppermint	Analgesic, antiseptic; vapor therapy useful in treatment of cold and cough
Pine	Disinfectant
Rose	Perfume, aromatherapeutic
Rosemary	Aromatherapeutic
Rosewood	Mild analgesic, antidepressant; vapor therapy useful for treatment of headache
Sandalwood	Soap and perfume; used in Ayurvedic medicine
Tea tree	Antibacterial; good for topical application
Thyme	Antibacterial; treats muscle pain, eczema
Ylang-ylang	Calming, fragrance
Wintergreen	Analgesic; can be fatal if ingested, oil not to be used as an aromatherapeutic

Antibacterial Properties of Essential Oils

Ancient Egyptians used aromatic plants in embalming to stop bacterial growth and decay; the antibacterial properties of these plants are attributed to their essential oils. Scientific studies indicate that essential oils act against a wide spectrum of pathogenic bacteria. Those oils with high concentrations of carvacrol and thymol (oregano, thyme, and savory oil) inhibit growth of many bacteria. Tea-tree oil has significant antibacterial properties, and unlike hand washes with antiseptic agents that may damage skin, tea-tree oil does not harm skin or affect its protective bacteria.[14] A cream formulary containing 10 percent tea-tree oil caused significant and fast relief against localized and acute dermatitis in dogs, compared with commercial skin-care cream.[15] However, tea-tree oil is very toxic if ingested and should be applied only topically. Tea-tree oil is also useful in treating mild skin rashes. I personally used tea-tree oil when I had a minor skin rash, and the rash resolved in three days. However, if the rash does not disappear or gets worse, you should consult your doctor to determine if you need a referral to a dermatologist.

Prabuseenivasan et al. studied the antibacterial effects of twenty-one essential oils and observed that nineteen of them had some efficacy against the organisms tested. Cinnamon, lime, geranium, rosemary, orange, lemon, and clove oil showed the maximum activity against all four g-negative bacteria tested and against two g-positive bacteria. Cinnamon oil showed the best antibacterial effect, and its active component, cinnamaldehyde also has antioxidant properties. Cinnamon oil is not harmful even if consumed with food products.[16] Essential oils can be incorporated into mouthwash or rinses for oral health. A six-month, controlled clinical study demonstrated that a mouthwash containing essential oil (Listerine Antiseptic, containing a fixed combination of essential oils as active ingredients; 0.064 percent thymol, 0.092 percent eucalyptol, 0.060 percent methyl salicylate, and 0.042 percent menthol) was equally effective in preventing dental plaque and gingivitis as was the synthetic antibacterial agent chlorhexidine.[17] Another study reported that peppermint oil and rosemary oil are superior to chlorhexidine in preventing dental biofilm formation by bacteria.[18] Common essential oils with antibacterial properties are listed in Table 3.3.

Essential oils and extracts also protect foods from spoilage bacteria and have been used for thousands of years in food preservation. Cinnamon, clove, and rosemary oil have strong and consistent activities against many pathogens.[19] In one study, the authors found that basil, lemon balm, marjoram, oregano, rosemary,

TABLE 3.3: Pharmacological Activities of Various Essential Oils

PHARMACOLOGICAL ACTIVITY	ESSENTIAL OIL
Antibacterial	Cilantro, cinnamon, clove, coriander, eucalyptus, geranium, lemon, lime, orange, oregano, peppermint, rosemary, savory, tea tree, thyme, sage
Antioxidant	Basil, cinnamon, clove, nutmeg, oregano, thyme
Antiviral	Anise, dwarf pine, chamomile, lemongrass, peppermint, tea tree
Aromatherapy	Basil, bergamot, cedarwood, chamomile, geranium, jasmine, lavender, rosemary, peppermint, rosewood, ylang-ylang
Preventing heart disease	Basil, cinnamon, cumin, garlic, oregano

sage, and thyme oils have significant activities against food-borne pathogens. Oregano and thyme oils showed the best effects against bacterial growth, and in combination they produced additional activities. The combinations of oregano with marjoram and thyme with sage showed the most promising results against *E. coli*.[20] Gutierrez et al. also demonstrated that on a carrot model product, basil, lemon balm, marjoram, oregano, and thyme were deemed organoleptically acceptable (did not alter taste, color, odor, or texture), but only oregano and marjoram essential oils were acceptable for lettuce.[21]

Antiviral Properties of Essential Oils

The herpes simplex virus (types 1 and 2) causes some of the most common infections in humans. Lemongrass essential oil possesses very potent action against herpes simplex virus-1, while peppermint oil demonstrates a high level of antiviral activity against herpes virus-2. Tea-tree oil and, to a lesser extent, eucalyptus oil also demonstrate activity against herpes virus-2.[22] Anise oil, dwarf pine oil, and chamomile oil also have activities against both acyclovir-sensitive and acyclovir-resistant herpes simplex virus type-1 strains.[23]

Antioxidant Properties of Essential Oils

Essential oils of basil, cinnamon, clove, nutmeg, oregano, and thyme have proven antioxidant capacities, with clove oil demonstrating the highest antioxidant capability. The antioxidant properties of these oils come from various active components, including phenolic compounds, terpene alcohols, ketones, and aldehydes.[24] In addition to its antioxidant capacity, clove oil also has significant activity against fungal infections, such as those caused by species of candida. Rosemary, eucalyptus, ylang-ylang, rose, parsley-seed, jasmine, and juniper-berry oils also have significant antioxidant effects. In one study, ylang-ylang, rose, parsley-seed, jasmine, and celery-seed oils showed significantly more antioxidant capacity than peppermint, chamomile, sandalwood, ginger, lavender, and angelica-seed oil.[25]

Essential Oils in Aromatherapy

Aromatherapy, the therapeutic use of essential oils through skin absorption or inhalation, was used in ancient Chinese medicine and Indian Ayurvedic medicine. Although *aromatherapy* refers to the action of aromatic compounds present in essential oils, other components in the oils may also be responsible for the therapeutic action. Ancient Egyptians used aromatic oils for perfumes. Scientific research demonstrates that inhaled or dermally applied essential oils enter the bloodstream and exert their beneficial effects as measured in cellular and animal models. In the United States, aromatherapy has been accepted as a legitimate part of holistic nursing.[26] Clinical studies have demonstrated reduced agitation in patients with dementia following lavender oil vaporization. Moreover, the sedative effect of lavender oil was evidenced by increased sleep time in dementia patients in residential care.[27] Another study noted significant reductions in disturbed behavior of ten dementia patients treated over a six-month period with a range of essential oils (vaporized mixtures of orange, ylang-ylang, patchouli, basil, rosemary, peppermint, rosewood, geranium, bergamot, chamomile, and jasmine). As a result, psychoactive medicines were reduced in a majority of these patients, causing overall cost savings and fewer side effects.[28]

Lavender essential oil is effective in treating sleep disorders and is a safe alternative to sleep medication. In one study, using a blend of basil, juniper, lavender, and sweet marjoram for massage was effective in increasing the sleep time of patients. Lavender oil is also effective in reducing anxiety. Chamomile oil helped in elevating the mood of subjects.[29] There are many published studies evaluating the effectiveness of aromatherapy massage in pain and anxiety control in various patient groups. Although results are mixed, in general there is a short-term benefit of aromatherapy massage in controlling depression and anxiety and elevating mood. However, care must be exercised in blending the right amount of essential oil with carrier oil for aromatherapy massage. Essential oils of citrus origin should be avoided due to known photosensitivity of the skin after application. In addition, only oils recommended by herbalists for aromatherapy should be used because certain essential oils can trigger allergic reactions.

Essential Oils and Cardiovascular Disease

Although results are mixed and several studies have shown that garlic oil does not significantly lower total cholesterol, in general it is accepted based on other studies that garlic reduces total cholesterol and helps to increase "good" (HDL or high-density lipoprotein) cholesterol.[30] In addition, garlic may also lower blood pressure in patients with elevated systolic blood pressure.[31] Garlic also has a strong antioxidant effect, which is beneficial in reducing the risk for cardiovascular disease. Hypertension is one of the risk factors for developing cardiovascular disease, including atherosclerosis, as well renal failure, eye disease (hypertensive retinopathy can cause serious problems including blindness), and a variety of other diseases. Oral administration of oregano, cinnamon, cumin, and other essential oils decreased blood pressures in rats. Essential oil of basil also lowers blood pressure.[32]

Miscellaneous Other Benefits of Essential Oils

Evening-primrose oil is high in linoleic acid, gamma-linolenic acid, and vitamin E. Consumption of evening-primrose oil appears to be safe with a few side effects: nausea, softening of stool, and headache. It also appears that evening-primrose oil offers benefits in treating atopic eczema and may have beneficial effects for patients with rheumatoid arthritis. Massage with aromatic ginger and orange essential oil is effective in reducing moderate to severe knee pain among elderly patients.[33]

Essential Oils with GRAS Status

The following essential oils have been granted GRAS (generally regarded as safe for human consumption) status by the FDA:

basil	bergamot
chamomile	cinnamon
citronella	clove
eucalyptus	garlic
grapefruit	hyssop
jasmine	lavender
lemon	mandarin orange

- nutmeg
- orange
- peppermint
- pine
- rose
- rosemary
- sandalwood
- tangerine
- thyme
- turmeric

Toxicity of Essential Oils

Many essential oils, such as tea tree and orange as well as certain oils frequently used in aromatherapy, can produce allergic reactions, especially in people who are prone to allergic reactions or those who have asthma. A single essential oil may contain forty or more components that undergo complex metabolic processes in the body, and more rigorous research is needed to fully evaluate which essential oils are truly safe for human applications. In general, with few exceptions, essential oils can provide many beneficial effects if used in small quantities for topical application or as an air freshener. Nutmeg ingested in large amounts produces hallucinations. Cinnamon oil may cause dermatitis; eucalyptus oil and wormwood oil, if ingested in toxic quantities, may cause seizure; pennyroyal oil has known hepatic toxicity and can even cause death; and peppermint oil may produce irregular breathing.[34] Ingestion of as little as 10 mL of clove oil can cause liver damage, but such toxicity can be treated with N-acetylcysteine.[35]

Fish Oil

Fish oil supplementation and the inclusion of fish in one's regular diet have proven beneficial effects. An interest in the therapeutic benefit of fish consumption came after a 1976 report that showed that high consumption of fish oil in Eskimos living in Greenland was associated with a decreased risk of cardiovascular disease. In that trial, using 11,324 patients, it was shown that fish diets provided significant reductions in all causes of mortality from cardiovascular disease within a study period of three-and-a-half years.[36] A recent study by Leon et al., which reviewed data from 30,000 patients, also concluded that fish oil supplementation was associated with a significant reduction in deaths from cardiac causes.[37] Although the link between omega-3 fatty acids and reduction in cardiovascular risks has not been well established, scientific research has clearly demonstrated that fish oil reduces serum triglyceride levels (high triglyceride is a risk for cardiovascular disease), reduces risk of sudden death from cardiac arrhythmias, decreases formation of atherosclerotic plaque on arterial walls, and may slightly reduce blood pressure.

The American Heart Association recommends eating fish (particularly fatty fish) at least two times a week. Fish is also a good source of protein and, unlike meats, it does not contain saturated fats. Fish oil supplements prepared from oily fish are rich in omega-3 fatty acids such as eicosapentaenoic acid and docosahexaenoic acid. Usually, predatory fish such as mackerel, flounder, salmon, tuna, and swordfish have higher amounts of omega-3 fatty acids in their tissue because their bodies have accumulated acids from prey fish. The American Heart Association also recommends that patients with cardiovascular disease take about 1 g per day of combined eicosapentaenoic acid and docosahexaenoic acid, preferably from fatty fish or fish oil capsules, in consultation with a physician. Patients required to lower their triglycerides should consume 2–4 g of fatty acids from fish per day, provided as capsules under a physician's care.[38]

Although fish oil supplements can lower triglycerides in diabetic patients, fish oil has no beneficial effect in controlling blood sugar. However, the benefits of fish oil supplements in relieving pain in patients with rheumatoid arthritis are well established, and the supplements are safer than the NSAIDs used in pain control. The anti-inflammatory effects of fish oil are linked to the production of alternative prostaglandins and the reduction in production of proinflammatory cytokines. Fish oil has another safety advantage in reducing cardiovascular risk factors in these patients because patients with rheumatoid arthritis are at higher risk of developing cardiovascular disease.[39]

Safety Considerations of Fish and Fish Oil

It has been suggested that the ingestion of fish oil can theoretically increase the risk of bleeding, but clinical studies have not shown any direct correlation. Although the combination of a small dose of aspirin (81 mg) and fish oil supplement may slightly increase bleeding time, the combination is usually considered safe. In contrast, patients receiving warfarin therapy (Coumadin) may be at higher risk of bleeding if they also consume significant amounts of fish oil daily. Buckley et al. observed that fish oil provided additional anticoagulation therapy when used with warfarin, and when a patient taking aspirin doubled her daily intake of fish oil supplement, her bleeding time, measured by a complex parameter called INR (international normalization ratio), was significantly increased, thus raising her risk of bleeding from warfarin therapy.[40]

> *Patients receiving warfarin therapy should consult with their physician before initiating daily intake of fish-oil supplement.*

Consumption of large amounts of fish may cause adverse results due to environmental contaminants such as organic and inorganic mercury (methyl mercury in particular), polychlorinated biphenyl (PCBs, used in a variety of products—production was banned in 1979 in the United States due to toxicity), and dioxins, which may also be present in fish, especially predatory fish. Pregnant women, women planning to become pregnant, and children should not eat fish (shark, swordfish, king mackerel, golden bass, and golden snapper) in which high amounts of mercury could accumulate. Other people can eat up to 7 oz of these fish per week. Salmon, cod, flounder, catfish, and other seafood such as crabs and scallops may also contain mercury but in lower amounts.[41] Contamination in certain brands of fish oil from these pollutants are reduced through purification. Consumers should be aware of this fact when selecting a brand of fish oil.[42] Fish-oil capsules, if left on the shelf for a prolonged time, may undergo oxidation. It is important to examine the manufacturing data and expiration date of fish-oil supplements and not to consume any fish-oil capsule after the expiration date. Try to find a product that has been freshly manufactured.

Recently, the FDA granted fish oil GRAS (generally regarded as safe for human consumption) status.

Conclusion

Essential oils and fish oils offer many benefits. Many of the benefits of essential oils are available through aromatherapy. Fish oils and many essential oils are considered safe supplements. However, as with any complementary and alternative therapy, it is advised that you inform your doctor that you are taking fish-oil supplement or using essential oils. You should not take any essential oil as a dietary supplement without consulting a qualified herbalist. Moreover, be sure to obtain your doctor's approval before taking any essential oils as a dietary supplement so you can avoid potential interactions with any other medications you are taking.

CHAPTER 4

Herbal Supplements That May Boost Your Immune System

At least eight hundred species of bacteria inhabit the human host, either on the skin or inside the body, representing a total population approaching 10^{15} organisms (1,000 trillion or 1 quadrillion). Put into perspective, the number of bacteria is far greater than the number of cells in our bodies. Organisms colonize various body tissues, representing species that take advantage of space and nutrients to coexist with us. However, under some conditions, this symbiotic relationship can produce disease. Combine that with the introduction of outside pathogens, such as those responsible for the common cold or flu, and it is easy to see why it is critical to keep our immune systems in peak order. For example, the common cold is the leading cause of visits to doctors' offices in the United States, accounting for 189 million lost school days. Influenza is a leading cause of morbidity and mortality, accounting for 20 to 25 million doctors' office visits per year and approximately 36,000 deaths.[1] Therefore, it is critical that we maintain a healthy immune response and even augment that response when warranted. Many of us try to boost our immune system by eating a proper diet and sometimes by taking herbal supplements. Among the supplements that have immune-boosting potential are:

- astragalus
- elderberry
- garlic
- goldenseal
- hyssop
- larch arabinogalactans
- olive leaf extract
- peppermint
- echinacea
- eucalyptus
- ginseng (Asian, North American, Siberian)
- honey
- isatis
- licorice
- osha
- sage

The Immune System

The immune system is an intricate network of cells, tissues, and organs that protects us from pathogens such as viruses, bacteria, and fungi. It can be weakened by multiple factors, from stress to nutrient deficiency to coinfection by other microbes in our bodies. Indeed, it is apparent that when there is a "hole" in our immune repertoire, such as that seen in patients with immunodeficiency or HIV infection, there is a weakening of the body's immune response, making individuals more susceptible to disease.

Herbal supplements hold the promise of strengthening our immune status, increasing our chance of fighting off infectious agents. Specifically, herbal supplements have demonstrated great benefit in multiple areas, including the ability to control inflammation, to boost innate responses to bacteria and other infectious agents, to moderate allergic reactions, and to regulate continuing autoimmune-related symptoms. The following short overview of basic immune function and the defense against pathogens will place the use of herbal supplements into perspective.

The first line of defense against pathogens is our skin and the mucous membranes that line our respiratory, gastrointestinal, and urinary tracts. These mucosal surfaces are rich in active cells, such as macrophages and neutrophils, that can trap pathogens and produce a local inflammatory response that is necessary to begin the clearance of the invading organism. This inflammatory response is beneficial and, in most cases, allows the establishment of an environment that activates a secondary level of cells (an adaptive immune response) to specifically fight the invading organisms. However, if these initial responses are not held in check, they can cause local tissue damage.

The secondary adaptive response recognizes foreign organisms using specific cell-surface receptors. This response is regulated by white blood cells known as lymphocytes, specifically the B and T lymphocytes produced in the bone marrow, which work in concert with macrophages (a type of white blood cell that ingests foreign objects, such as pathogenic bacterial cells, in order to neutralize them) at the site of infection. The B lymphocytes make antibodies, complex proteins of high molecular weight (also called immunoglobulins) that stick to and tag the foreign pathogen for subsequent destruction and elimination. The B lymphocytes are assisted in making antibodies through the action of the T lymphocytes, which serve as ringleaders in controlling the overall immune function by way of released chemical mediators, called cytokines. In many cases, herbal supplements can help to modulate which chemical mediators or cytokines are released, either from the T lymphocytes or from the macrophage population, so as to direct or modulate the response in a productive manner.

The activity of herbal supplements in mediating immune function can be a powerful tool in the fight against pathogens. The same is true for modulation of responses that occur in other deleterious immune reactions. For example, allergies develop when the immune process is triggered by a harmless, everyday foreign object such as dust, pollen, or animal dander. Inhaled or ingested allergens produce an immediate allergic reaction (hypersensitivity), resulting from a specific subset of antibodies that recognizes these foreign particles and subsequently triggers mast cells (a connective tissue cell whose normal function is not fully understood) to release many molecules, most notably histamine, which binds through the employment of histamine receptors, triggering the allergic reaction. Allergy medicines (antihistamines) inhibit the combination of histamine with histamine receptors, thus relieving us of an allergic reaction. Many herbal supplements have been proven to moderate this response, thus alleviating symptoms associated with the allergic reaction.

In a similar manner, autoimmune responses arise when our bodies mistakenly identify parts of ourselves as foreign. This response is always mediated by the reactivity of B and T lymphocytes, or by a combination of the two working in concert. Herbal supplements have the potential to mediate these responses as well, mostly by limiting the exaggeration of effects and thus lowering overall destructive self-reactivity.

Finally, proper nutrition is essential in maintaining a healthy immune system. Nutrients such as vitamins, folic acid, and minerals are necessary for immune-system function. Deficiency of even a single nutritional element such as iron, copper, zinc, selenium, vitamins A, B_6, C, E, and folic acid can reduce immune surveillance and response to pathogenic agents.

Of the herbal supplements that may boost the immune system, many, such as astragalus, echinacea, elderberry, ginseng, goldenseal, and olive leaf, help to prevent the common cold and flu. Others, such as licorice and sage, are instrumental in modifying inflammation. Overall, when used appropriately, these herbal supplements have the potential to direct immune responses away from harmful disorders.

Astragalus

Traditionally, astragalus was used in Chinese medicine, usually in combination with other herbs, to stimulate the immune system. It is still used in China to treat hepatitis and as an adjunct therapy for cancer. In the United States, people take this herbal supplement mostly as an immune stimulant in order to prevent the common cold and upper respiratory infections. There is also a popular belief that astragalus is useful in treating heart disease. Typically, roots of astragalus are used for preparing an extract or for brewing a tea mixture. Astragalus is also used in combination with other herbs such as licorice, ginseng, and angelica.

Research has indicated that in mice astragalus can stimulate immune function and rejuvenate depressed immune function.[2] In one study conducted in China, sixty-two patients with congestive heart failure were divided into two groups. One group received 30 mL of astragalus injection, while the other group received a nitroglycerin injection (10 mg). In the patients who received astragalus, clinical heart function improved significantly, as did markers of improved immune function. The authors concluded that astragalus can be used as an auxiliary treatment for congestive heart failure.[3] Also, because astragalus is capable of stimulating the immune system, it may be effective in preventing cold and other infections.

Astragalus has been shown to have anticancer properties. In one study, the authors demonstrated the antitumor activity of astragalus against human colon-cancer cells and hepatocellular carcinoma (liver-cancer) cells.[4] Astragalus can also restore impaired T-cell function in cancer patients. The antitumor effect may be achieved through activation of the antitumor immune mechanism of the cancer patient. A few studies have indicated the benefit of using astragalus along with other herbs as an adjunct therapy for cancer patients, but these studies, in general, are not well designed.

The polysaccharide molecules found in astragalus can prevent diabetes, according to studies using mice. Astragalus is generally considered a safe and effective herbal supplement.

Echinacea

Echinacea, a genus including nine species, is a member of the daisy family. Three species, *Echinacea angustifolia*, *Echinacea pallida*, and *Echinacea purpurea*, are found in common herbal preparations. Native Americans considered this plant to be a blood purifier. Today, echinacea is used mainly as an immune stimulant in order to increase resistance to colds, influenza, and other infections, and it is one of the most popular herbs in the United States. The fresh herb, freeze-dried herb, and alcoholic extract are all commercially available. The aerial part of the plant (the part that is above ground) and fresh or dried root can also be used to prepare echinacea tea. One of the constituents of echinacea, arabinogalactan, may have immune-boosting capacity, as was discovered in a study using an animal model.[5] Other studies using cellular models have demonstrated that echinacea preparations can stimulate the immune system, but clinical studies using human subjects have returned mixed results. Some studies failed to demonstrate any beneficial effect of echinacea in preventing cold or flu, while others reported positive findings.

Study by our research group demonstrated that in mouse spleen cells, echinacea extract was able to stimulate production of interleukins and other markers of immune stimulation in these cells. The water extract of echinacea was more effective than pure alcohol extract in stimulating immune reaction.[6] Sullivan et al. reported that on the cellular level, echinacea extract stimulates macrophages to produce interleukins, tumor necrosis factor, and nitrous oxide, thus providing evidence of the immune-stimulatory capability of echinacea extract. Moreover, the authors observed that oral administration of echinacea extract can reduce the bacterial count of the bacteria *Listeria monocytogenes*.[7]

However, some clinical studies using human subjects did not observe any protective effect of echinacea against a cold. The ability of oral echinacea preparation to delay the onset of an upper respiratory infection was compared with that of a placebo in 302 volunteers from an industrial plant and several military institutions. Although subjects felt significantly better after taking echinacea, rigorous statistical analysis did not show any significant benefit in delaying the onset of upper-respiratory-tract infection.[8] In another report, the authors evaluated data from three clinical studies and concluded that the likelihood of experiencing symptoms of cold was 55 percent higher in subjects who received placebo than in subjects who received echinacea supplement. The authors concluded that echinacea extract is capable of preventing symptoms of the common cold after clinical inoculation by cold viruses.[9]

Data from clinical studies and other reporting programs indicate that adverse reactions from use of echinacea are not common. Common side effects are gastrointestinal upset and rashes; in rare cases, echinacea may be associated with severe allergic reaction. Short-term use of echinacea is safe with only a slight risk of adverse effects. However, data indicates that pregnant women and nursing mothers probably should avoid its use.[10]

Elderberry

Elderberry (*Sambucus nigra*) is a plant of the honeysuckle family. Extract of the berries has been traditionally used for treating cold and flu symptoms and conditions, and it contains many ingredients, including rutin, anthocyanin, quercetin, and flavonoids. Research has demonstrated that elderberry extract acts against influenza A, influenza B, and herpes simplex virus. Elderberry anthocyanin flavonoids also have antioxidant properties. In a clinical study involving sixty patients (aged eighteen to fifty-four) suffering from influenza-like symptoms for forty-eight hours or less, one group of patients received 15 mL of elderberry syrup (1 tbsp) four times a day for five days, while another group received a placebo. In the treatment group, the majority of patients reported significant improvement of symptoms in three to four days, but the group that received the placebo took seven to eight days before their conditions improved. The authors concluded that elderberry extract seems to offer an efficient, cost-effective, and safe treatment for influenza.[11] Elderberry syrup is also sold under the trade name Sambucol. Elder tree leaf is on the GRAS list, but elderberries are not.

Eucalyptus Oil

Eucalyptus oil has long been recognized for its antibacterial and anti-inflammatory potential. Topical ointment containing eucalyptus oil has been used traditionally to heal wounds and treat fungal infection, and tea prepared from eucalyptus has been used in reducing fever. Eucalyptus oil also has expectorant properties and may be useful in relieving symptoms of cold and flu. Scientific research has shown that eucalyptus oil is capable of boosting immunity.[12] Eucalyptus oil is safe and is on the GRAS list.

Garlic

Garlic, as discussed in Chapter 2, offers many health benefits, including help in preventing cold and flu symptoms by boosting the immune system. It also has anticancer and antioxidant properties. The odor-producing allicin in garlic can be eliminated and modified by extraction with alcohol, wine, milk, vinegar, or soy sauce, and such extracts retain many of garlic's beneficial effects. Although it was long thought that allicin was responsible for garlic's many beneficial actions, recent research has shown that other components of garlic also have substantial medicinal value. Aged garlic extract is an antioxidant and is used for preventing colds.[13] Josling used forty-six volunteers who took either allicin-containing garlic extract or placebo over a period of twelve weeks between November and February and concluded that the subjects who took garlic supplement had significantly fewer colds than the placebo group. Moreover, in the case of colds, the subjects who took a garlic supplement recovered faster than the placebo group. Therefore, an allicin-containing garlic supplement can prevent an attack by the common cold virus.[14] Garlic is a safe and effective herbal supplement and is on the GRAS list.

Ginseng

Asian ginseng (*Panax ginseng*) is primarily used to improve psychological function and exercise performance, to boost immune function, and to lower blood sugar in diabetes patients. Ginseng may also be effective in treating erectile dysfunction and in lowering the risk of cancer. Other uses of ginseng were discussed in Chapter 2; here we will address the effectiveness of ginseng in stimulating the immune system. Scientific studies have documented the immune-stimulatory capacity of Asian ginseng. A study involving 227 healthy volunteers showed that daily administration of 100 mg of ginseng extract enhanced the efficacy of influenza vaccine. The patients who received ginseng had a lower incidence of influenza and colds.[15] Another study, involving sixty volunteers with acute bronchitis, found that patients who were treated with both an antibiotic and ginseng had faster recoveries and their infections cleared faster than patients who received only antibiotics.

Extracts of North American ginseng (also known as American ginseng; *Panax quinquefolium*) have been found to have potential to modulate both natural and acquired immune response. In one clinical study, researchers looked at the effectiveness of North American ginseng in preventing a cold virus infection in 323 subjects with a history of at least two colds in the previous year. Some subjects dropped out of the study. Eventually data was obtained from 130 volunteers who took two capsules of North American ginseng for four months and from 149 subjects who took a placebo. Data showed that subjects who took the ginseng had significantly fewer episodes of colds compared with the placebo group. Moreover, the number of days the subjects suffered from a cold in a four-month period was lower in the ginseng group (mean 10.8 days) compared with the placebo group (mean cold days: 16.5).[16] Siberian ginseng may also stimulate the immune system. However, some preparations of imported Asian and Siberian ginseng may be contaminated with herbs and may not contain sufficient active ingredients. Ginseng supplements made by American-based companies may be more standardized. Ginseng is a relatively expensive supplement, and you should research the supplement manufacturer's quality-control practices before purchasing it.

Goldenseal

Goldenseal is a small plant native to North America that produces raspberry-like fruit. The root was used by Native Americans as a clothing dye and also for treating inflammation and infection of the eyes and skin. Goldenseal extract—from the root of the plant—is used today for relieving symptoms of cold and flu, sore throat, and canker sores, as well as for treating a variety of other conditions such as ulcer, mild eye irritation, and indigestion. Goldenseal is a very popular dietary supplement in the United States, especially in combination with echinacea for preventing cold and flu, and is one of the fifteen top-selling herbal supplements today.

The bioactivity of goldenseal is mainly due to the activity of the plant alkaloids berberine, hydrastine, and canadine. In a study using a mouse model, berberine was capable of stimulating production of interleukin, indicating that it may be useful in treating allergic disease.[17] Berberine also acts against various parasites such as tapeworm, viruses, and candida (yeast) infection; it is known to stimulate the immune system. Rehman et al. reported that like echinacea, goldenseal has immune-boosting effects as evidenced by an increase in primary immunoglobulin response (IGM) against an antigen in rats. (An antigen is a substance that causes an immune reaction; for example, an antigen can be a foreign object such as pollen that may cause allergy or a bacteria or virus.) The authors concluded that goldenseal enhances immune response by increasing specific immunoglobulin production against the antigen.[18]

Goldenseal is a slow-growing plant, and roots are harvested three to five years after planting. Because it takes so long to grow this herb, a dishonest manufacturer may "cut" the goldenseal preparation with other herbs such as yellow root, celandine, barberry, and Oregon grape, which also contain berberine. However, these contaminated products may not actually contain goldenseal or they may not contain the active components hydrastine and canadine. It has been reported that goldenseal may reduce the effectiveness of certain antibiotics, such as dioxyline, so if you are taking antibiotics, it may be wise not to use goldenseal.

Honey

Honey has been used since ancient times by the Egyptians, Romans, and Greeks. This natural sweetener was so highly regarded in Egyptian and Indian culture that it was included in offerings to the gods. The therapeutic uses of honey include treating wounds, ulcers, tonsillitis, gum disease, and fungal and bacterial infection. Clinical trials have established honey's antibacterial and wound-healing properties.[19] Honey is also used traditionally to treat cold and flu. My grandmother treated me with honey and extract of tulsi (Holy Basil) leaves (the tulsi plant grows naturally throughout India and is considered sacred by Hindus) whenever I got a cold. A recent publication confirms my grandmother's wisdom and shows that honey enhances the immune system and thus is helpful in treating colds. In addition, honey has antitumor and wound-healing properties.[20] Honey is a safe and effective supplement.

Hyssop

Hyssop (*Hyssop officinalis*) originated in the Black Sea area in central Asia. Its fragrant flowers and leaves are used for making extract, which is a popular herbal supplement during the winter months for preventing cold and flu and for relieving chest congestion and cold symptoms. It also contains a volatile oil, which may provide cold relief when inhaled. Hyssop is considered safe and is on the GRAS list. At this point, claims of hyssop relieving symptoms of cold and flu have not been verified by rigorous human clinical trials.

Larch Arabinogalactans

Larch arabinogalactan supplement is prepared from the wood of the Western larch tree and is indicated for stimulating the immune system. It is also a source of dietary fiber. Research has shown that larch arabinogalactans enhance the immune system and may be an effective adjunct for treating colds and flu.[21] These compounds are readily soluble in water. Larch arabinogalactan is safe and is on the GRAS list.

Licorice

Licorice, discussed in detail in Chapter 2, is believed to have immune-boosting effects. In Japan, licorice extract has been used for more than sixty years to treat chronic hepatitis C infection. Clinical trials have indicated that licorice extract can lower liver enzymes, which are markers of liver damage, in the blood of patients infected with hepatitis C. Aqueous extract of licorice can strengthen immune function by enhancing the production of interleukin by macrophages. It also has antiviral activity against herpes simplex virus type 1, influenza virus, and cytomegalovirus and can inhibit replication of HIV.[22] Glycyrrhizin, the active component of licorice root, is effective in reducing morbidity and mortality in mice infected with lethal doses of influenza virus.[23] Licorice may also help in weight loss. Several studies have shown that licorice may also have anticancer properties.

Licorice is a safe and effective herbal supplement and is on the FDA's GRAS list. However, it can increase blood pressure and thus should not be taken by individuals suffering from hypertension.

Olive Leaf

Olive-leaf extract has been used in folk medicine for centuries for treating colds and flu. It contains oleuropein, which has potent antibacterial, anti-inflammatory, and antioxidant properties. Other complex compounds found in olive-leaf extract can be effective against the influenza virus and certain bacteria. Scientific studies suggest that components of olive-leaf extract can reduce the infectivity of viruses that cause colds, influenza, and related infections. For a sore throat, gargling with olive-leaf extract may relieve symptoms by decreasing inflammation.[24] The extract is generally considered safe for short-term use; long-term safety has not been established.

Osha

Osha is a medical plant used in popular folk remedies in Mexico. The root is believed to boost immune function, prevent colds, and treat sore throat, and osha tea is used for relief of cold symptoms. At this point, no rigorous clinical human trials have confirmed the efficacy of osha root in preventing colds and flu.

Peppermint Oil

Peppermint oil is used for multiple purposes and is effective in stimulating the immune system. Menthol found in peppermint has a soothing effect on sore throats. Peppermint extract is also clinically effective in alleviating the nasal symptoms of allergic rhinitis.[25] Peppermint is safe and is on the GRAS list.

Sage

Of the many species of sage, *Salvia officinalis,* also known as common sage, is used for its medicinal properties. (Note: The *Salvia divinorum* plant contains dangerous psychoactive compounds and should never be used.) In traditional Chinese medicine, sage was used to increase physical strength and to enhance breast-milk production in women. Sage leaf was also used traditionally to treat sore throat and inflammation of the gums, and today a topical preparation of sage leaf is available for treating gum infections. This product should be gargled with as recommended but not swallowed.

Besides being used as a culinary spice, sage has also been used traditionally as an antiseptic, an anti-inflammatory, and a calming agent. Fresh sage leaves contain a variety of important active ingredients such as saponins and flavonoids as well as vitamins C and A. Sage tea has a soothing, antiseptic effect on mucus and is recommended for relieving congestion and other symptoms of upper-respiratory-tract infection.

Sage also has antioxidant activity.[26] Animal studies indicate that it may lower blood glucose and therefore may be beneficial for diabetics. Sage is a safe and effective herb and is on the GRAS list. However, pregnant women should not use sage without approval from their clinician.

Other Miscellaneous Agents

Both the leaves and roots of isatis (*Isatis tinctoria*), or woad, have been used for treatment of various infections including upper-respiratory-tract infection, influenza, and gastroenteritis. The antimicrobial action of the root is similar to that of berberine (see under "Goldenseal"). Isatis may be capable of increasing immune function. An herbal formula containing dry ivy-leaf extract as the main ingredient, in combination with thyme, aniseed, and marshmallow root, was effective in reducing cough in a clinical trial involving sixty-two patients who ingested 10 mL of the cough syrup for twelve days. The syrup was well tolerated, and the authors concluded that it was effective in alleviating cough in patients with colds, bronchitis, or respiratory-tract infection.[27]

Conclusion

Several herbal supplements are available for combating infectious agents such as those that cause the common cold and flu. Indeed, supplements such as echinacea and goldenseal are among the most popular herbal supplements sold today. Short-term use of most of these supplements is safe, and scientific research indicates that some of these are effective in boosting immune function, through control of inflammatory response, quieting allergic reactions, or regulating autoimmune function. Some may even be beneficial to prime the immune system so as to prevent attacks from viruses. Although many of the mechanisms underlying their usefulness are still under investigation, it is clear that herbal supplements hold promise to both moderate our responses against pathogens and speed recovery from infections.

CHAPTER 5

Homeopathic Remedies: Relatively Safe Alternative Medicine

Homeopathy is a form of complementary and alternative medicine that was introduced by Christian Friedrich Samuel Hahnemann (1755–1843), a German physician who received his medical degree in 1779. At that time, conventional medical treatments had no sound scientific basis; mainstream medicine focused on restoring balance by either "removing excess humor" (a "humor" was one of the four substances a body was thought to be made of, and which were thought to determine a person's health and character) or suppressing symptoms. Removing excess humor involved dangerous procedures such as bloodletting and purging the body using toxic substances, laxatives, enemas, giving patients nauseous substances so that they could vomit, and administration of complex mixtures such as Venice treacle, which was composed of sixty-four ingredients including opium and viper's flesh. Such procedures often worsened the symptoms and sometimes caused death.

Although trained in conventional medicine, Hahnemann became disillusioned with these medical practices and rejected many of them as irrational and dangerous. In 1789, when he was translating *A Treatise on Materia Medica,* an early book on pharmacology by the famous British professor of chemistry and medicine, Dr. William Cullen, into German, he first conceived the principles of homeopathy and decided to do experiments with cinchona bark, from which quinine was later derived. Hahnemann favored use of a single medicine in low dosages to treat a disease. Homeopathy is based on a vitalistic view of how the human body functions. Vitalism holds that a vital principle (which today may be called "energy") animates the body, and when all the vital powers of the body are in harmony a person is disease-free, but any imbalance results in sickness. In Hahnemann's opinion, a disease has both physical and spiritual causes and treatment should integrate mind and body. Homeopathy in that sense is a holistic medicine, sharing with traditional Chinese medicine, Indian Ayurveda, and other ancient forms of medicines the philosophy that the body has the capacity to heal itself and that the healing process requires participation of both mind and body in order to restore balance between the various vital forces of life.

In 1796 Hahnemann published his principles of homeopathy in "Essay on a New Principle of Ascertaining the Curative Power of Drugs"; this essay is considered the birth of homeopathy. In 1810 he published his groundbreaking book *The Organon of the Healing Art*.[1] The sixth edition of *Organon* was published in 1920, long after Hahnemann's death.[2]

A Brief History of Homeopathy in the United States

Homeopathy was introduced in the United States around 1825; Dr. Constantine Hering, who immigrated to the United States from Germany in 1833, is generally considered the father of American homeopathy. For the remainder of the nineteenth century, homeopathy gained tremendous popularity in the United States partly due to the lack of sound scientific theory as well as the lack of available medicines in conventional medical practice. Homeopathy was credited in both the United States and Europe with widespread success in dealing with a number of epidemics. Homeopathic practitioners claimed better results than their conventional colleagues for the treatment of epidemic cholera.

In 1831 the Asiatic cholera epidemic, which started in India, had spread to Europe. Hahnemann, receiving a detailed description of symptoms, was able to predict effective homeopathic remedies. His protocol for treating cholera included cleanliness, disinfection, and ventilation and resulted in between 2 to 20 percent mortality compared with over 50 percent mortality in patients who received conventional medical care. The Royal London Homeopathic Hospital, which played a vital role in treating patients during that city's cholera epidemic, is still in public service after 150 years and is evidence of the efficacy of homeopathy.[3]

Beginning in the mid-1800s homeopathy was taught side by side with conventional medicine in the United States. The first women's medical college in the United States, Boston Female Medical College, was founded in 1848, and professional homeopathic medical societies were the first to accept women physicians into their membership. Interestingly, the American Medical Association was formed after the foundation of American Institute of Homeopathy. In 1900 there were twenty-two homeopathic medical schools in the United States and more than one hundred homeopathic hospitals. During that time, one out of five practitioners incorporated homeopathy into medical practice. In 1903 the American Medical Association, after long antagonism, invited homeopaths to join its ranks.[4] However, following that alliance, more funding became available for conventional medical schools, and antagonism between conventional doctors and homeopathic practitioners resulted in a decrease in funding to homeopathic medical colleges. By 1923 the number of homeopathic medical colleges in the United States was reduced to only two. The homeopathic branch of the Hahnemann Medical School was closed in 1949.[5] However, in the rest of the world, homeopathy is taught in colleges and is sometimes integrated with conventional medical education. There are several colleges in the United Kingdom, continental Europe, and Australia that offer formal courses in homeopathy. In India there are more than one hundred colleges that train students in homeopathic medicine, which is recognized by the federal and state governments of India. More than twenty homeopathic colleges in India are government-run.

Because of public interest, in 1996 the European Parliament issued a mandate to the European Commission to investigate whether homeopathy was beneficial. Subsequently, the group recommended that homeopathy be integrated into all medical-school curricula. In 1998 the French Council called for official recognition of homeopathy by incorporating homeopathy into medical-school curricula. The Glasgow Homeopathic Hospital in Scotland is a part of the United Kingdom's National Health Service.[6]

Principles of Homeopathy

Homeopathy emphasizes the self-healing potential of the body and of mind-body integration. In the homeopathic view, an illness develops when there is an imbalance in the vital life forces. This is similar to the beliefs on which traditional Chinese medicine and ancient Indian Ayurvedic medicine are based. A remedy prescribed by a homeopathic practitioner is meant to correct the imbalance in the body and cure the illness. In addition, homeopathy has the following two core principles:

1. *"Similia similibus curantur,"* or "like cures like." If any compound or toxin

produces particular symptoms in a healthy individual, then that compound is capable of curing an individual who shows these symptoms.

2. The power of dilution. Hahnemann recognized that the use of a compound that produces a symptom in a healthy individual may aggravate symptoms of disease in a sick person. Therefore, he advocated dilution of the substance to a point where such symptoms are no longer present. In fact, in homeopathic medicine it is believed that medicines with higher dilutions are stronger and have a higher efficacy than the same medicines in lower dilutions.

These principles are discussed further below.

Similia Similibus Curantur ("Like Cures Like")

The major principle of homeopathy is that a doctor can cure a disease using a diluted form of a substance that would induce the symptoms of that disease in a healthy person. The word *homeopathy* is derived from the Greek word *omeos*, meaning "similar," and *pathos*, meaning "suffering." This is in sharp contrast with *allopathy*, which is derived from the Greek word *allo*, which means "different," and *pathos*. Hahnemann coined the term *allopathy* to describe how conventional medical practice differed from homeopathic practice. In allopathy, the objective of treatment is to interfere with or block a pathological process by which a disease can be cured or at least symptoms of a disease can be suppressed. (Interestingly, in immunization, a small dose of live or dead pathogen is injected into a healthy person so that person develops immunity against the disease—which is a homeopathic idea.) Hahnemann published *Essays on a New Principle for Ascertaining the Curative Power of Drugs* in 1796, the same year that Edward Jenner showed that giving individuals small doses of cowpox protected them against smallpox.[7] Although there was significant research in both homeopathy and allopathy in the 1800s, later allopathic medicine took a more successful route and became the foundation of modern Western medicine, the major form of health care worldwide. Unfortunately, homeopathic research lagged behind, and now homeopathy is considered a complementary and alternative medicine.

In the early days of his medical practice Hahnemann started taking regular dosages of cinchona bark (which contains quinine), which produced symptoms of malaria in him. From that experiment he got the idea of "*Similia similibus curantur*"—if an individual has an illness, then a medicine that produces similar symptoms in a healthy individual, administered in a smaller dose, should be able to cure the illness in the sick individual. Hahnemann called this process "proving," and he performed experiments on himself and his friends with many such medicines, including several toxic substances such as arsenic, mercury, and belladonna. He claimed to be able to compile a collection of applicable medicines, often termed homeopathic remedies. He cited Jenner's use of the cowpox vaccination to prevent smallpox as an example of the like-cures-like principle.[8] Similarly, bee stings trigger allergic reactions. Therefore, a homeopathic remedy prepared from honey-bees (*Apis mellifica*) should be effective in treating allergic reactions.[9] The homeopathic remedy *Allium cepa*, which is derived from onions, should be able to cure a cold, because in healthy people cutting onions induces teary eyes and runny nose, effects similar to the symptoms of the common cold.

Samuel Hahnemann's contributions to medicine are not limited to the foundation of homeopathy. He also helped to identify the clinical significance of many medicines, such as quinine and digitalis, which are still used in conventional Western medicines today.[10] He also advocated individualization of treatment based on the totality of a patient's symptoms in order to address the root cause of disease. He established that medicines should be given in a minimal quantity to treat a disease in order to avoid adverse reactions. These principles are all followed in today's practice of modern medicine and in "personalized medicine," which is geared toward finding a particular medicine in a specially adjusted dosage for an individual patient. Such practices may have a root in the concept preached by Hahnemann two hundred years ago.

The Power of Dilution

Early in his medical practice, Hahnemann recommended dosages comparable to those given by traditional medical practitioners, such as ½ grain (1 grain = 65 mg) of opium, 3.9 grains of cinchona, etc. Soon, however, he recognized the toxic effects of such high dosages and made a considerable change by diluting the medication. He developed a new way of preparing homeopathic remedies by a process known as dilution and succussion. If a particular compound is soluble in alcohol, then a "mother tincture" is prepared by dissolving that substance in alcohol. A drop of the mother tincture is then diluted with water, followed by vigorous shaking of the mixture (succussion). The preparation is then diluted further and further until the desired concentration is achieved. Finally, alcohol is added to the final dilution to preserve the remedy, and the remedy is sprayed over sugar pellets or may be used as a liquid preparation. As the pellets are dried, the alcohol evaporates.[11] There are two different ways of diluting the mother tincture, decimal dilution ($\frac{1}{10}$ dilution in each step, termed the *x* scale of dilution) and centesimal dilution ($\frac{1}{100}$ dilution in each step, termed the *c* scale). (See Table 5.1.)

TABLE 5.1: Homeopathic Dilution in Preparing Remedies

DILUTION	PROCESS
Mother tincture	Prepared following guidelines defined in the *Homeopathic Pharmacopeia of the United States*
1c	1 part mother tincture to 99 parts water
2c	1 part 1c dilution in 99 parts water
3c	1 part 2c dilution in 99 parts water
4c	1 part 3c dilution in 99 parts water
5c	1 part 4c dilution in 99 parts water
6c	1 part 5c dilution in 99 parts water
12c	1 part 11c dilution in 99 parts water*
Mother tincture	Prepared following guidelines defined in the *Homeopathic Pharmacopeia of the United States*
1x	1 part mother tincture to 9 parts water
2x	1 part 1x dilution in 9 parts water
3x	1 part 2x dilution in 9 parts water
4x	1 part 3x dilution in 9 parts water
5x	1 part 4x dilution in 9 parts water
6x	1 part 5x dilution in 9 parts water
24x	1 part 23x dilution in 9 parts water*

* At this dilution, Avogadro's number, beyond which no molecule can exist in the preparation, is reached.

Hahnemann observed that in the process of succussion, the medicinal properties of the substance were transferred to the molecules of water (this is called potentization). He explained that through this process, the toxic properties of a substance were diminished but its therapeutic potential was increased. A homeopathic remedy is administered at a particular potency (e.g., 6c, 30c), and at that extreme dilution, virtually no toxic side effect of a substance can persist. This is the reason homeopathic remedies are safe and rarely have side effects. However, in modern science, the efficacy of a homeopathic substance cannot be proven because there is no valid scientific explanation of the transfer of properties of a substance into molecules of water during vigorous shaking.

A variety of substances derived from plants, animals, minerals, and synthetics (chemicals produced by combining natural ingredients using a specific chemical process) are used in homeopathy. For example, *Natrum muriaticum* is table salt, while *Lachesis muta* is prepared from the venom of the bushmaster snake. Aconite is derived from the monkshood plant. Compounds that are not soluble in alcohol are incorporated in homeopathic remedies in a different way. In this process, a finely ground substance is mixed with lactose and ground with a pestle in a mortar. Then a portion of that mixture is diluted further with lactose. After six such processes, when 6x dilutions is reached, serial dilution with water can be carried out to reach the desired potency.

Other Principles of Homeopathy

For Hahnemann, the whole body and spirit was the focus of the treatment, and he routinely spent a great deal of time with his patients, asking them not only about their illness but also about their lifestyles. His gentle approach contrasted sharply with the harsh procedures employed by conventional medical practitioners. Hahnemann also believed that one medicine was capable of curing a disease, while his allopathic counterparts treated patients with a combination of active substances, including toxic substances. Therefore, patients never felt ill effects from homeopathic remedies, whereas during Hahnemann's lifetime, allopathic treatment could result in worsening of symptoms and even death.

In addition to the "vitalistic" approach, a principle called "miasm" also gained acceptance in homeopathy. *Miasm* means a supposed predisposition to a disease. Hahnemann noticed that certain patients had chronic tendencies toward certain diseases. These chronic tendencies, or miasms, are inherited, so if a homeopathic practitioner knows the miasm of a patient, they can treat the root cause of the disease, thus preventing it from developing. In this sense, Hahnemann intuitively understood about genetic predisposition to disease, a concept that is well accepted in modern medicine and enables physicians to try to prevent that disease by giving proper medication. For example, if high cholesterol is common among family members, then a cholesterol-lowering drug may be prescribed along with proper diet and exercise in order to keep the blood cholesterol level under control in an effort to prevent heart disease or a heart attack.

Another important principle of homeopathy is Hering's law of cure. According to Constantine Hering, healing begins in the deepest part of the organism, where the root of the disease resides, and progresses outward, where the more superficial symptoms are expressed. For example, when a homeopathic practitioner treats a child with asthma and eczema, it is expected that symptoms of asthma, such as wheezing, will disappear first, since these are deeper symptoms of the root cause of disease, followed by eczema, which is a more superficial symptom.[12]

Hahnemann claimed that homeopathy could cure virtually all diseases. However, his followers later modified that claim in order to gain more acceptance from conventional doctors. Hahnemann showed no interest in detailed pathology or in conventional diagnosis and treatment.[13]

Current Acceptance of Homeopathy in the United States

As described earlier, the popularity enjoyed by homeopathy in the nineteenth century in the United States began to decline at the beginning of the twentieth century. The Flexner Report of 1910, named for Abraham Flexner and sponsored by the American Medical Association, supported conventional medical-school training and condemned homeopathic schools. However, in as early as 1814 homeopathic practitioners had clashed with conventional medical practitioners. In 1842 Dr. Oliver Wendell Holmes, noted physician, poet, and humorist, ridiculed the approach of dilution (after the fourth dilution, the ratio of medicine to solution is 1 in 100 million parts water) when he said, "By the time the seventeenth degree of dilution should be reached, the alcohol required would equal in quantity the waters of ten thousand Adriatic seas." Hahnemann also certainly didn't help his cause by claiming in 1828 that all chronic diseases were caused by "the itch" (scabies, a red inflammation of the skin caused by mites).[14]

In the twentieth century, conventional medicine saw tremendous developments: the discovery of penicillin and many lifesaving drugs, new procedures for surgery, organ transplant, and the understanding of various diseases through detailed pathology. Unfortunately, homeopathy lagged behind in scientific research and the development of new remedies.

Despite these setbacks in the 1930s, homeopathy is now on the rise in the United States. The 1960s and 1970s saw a revival of homeopathy in many countries, and in 2002 the number of people in the United States using homeopathic remedies had increased by 500 percent over the previous seven years. The individuals using homeopathy tended to be affluent, white, and young.[15] Currently, there is no licensing for homeopathic practitioners in the United Sates, although courses of homeopathy are offered and certification is available. Many Doctors of Naturopathy (NDs) practice homeopathy under their license (several states grant holders of the ND degree a formal license to practice, but these licenses are not equivalent to medical licenses granted to Doctors of Medicine or Doctors of Osteopathic Medicine). Acupuncturists and chiropractors also sometimes practice homeopathy.[16]

Regulation of Homeopathic Remedies in the United States

Homeopathic remedies have been in use in the United States since 1835, but these remedies were not a part of the Food and Drug Act of 1906. However, when the act was revised in 1938, homeopathic remedies were included and became regulated by the FDA. In 1988 the FDA published guidelines under which homeopathic remedies could be sold legally, and most remedies are available over-the-counter. At present, more than twenty-five substances from plant, animal, and mineral sources are used in preparing homeopathic remedies.[17]

FDA regulation of homeopathic remedies is significantly different from that of conventional medicine. Manufacturers of homeopathic remedies are deferred from submitting new drug applications to the FDA, and their manufacturing processes are exempt from good manufacturing practice requirements for pharmaceutical companies, which include expiration dating of each product. Homeopathic remedies are sold in oral form or as creams for topical application. The label must state that the product is homeopathic and provide the name of the manufacturer. These remedies are not required to list all active ingredients and their strength (such as 6c) on the label, which is in contrast to pharmaceuticals, where it is mandatory to list all active ingredients and the amount(s) contained. The rationale for this exemption is that the concentration of an active ingredient in a homeopathic remedy is infinitely minute, thus there is no potential for toxicity.

Another difference is the amount of alcohol in homeopathic remedies. Conventional medicines for adults may not contain more than 10 percent alcohol, and the amount is even less for children's formulations. However, because alcohol is an integral part of homeopathic remedies, some preparations may contain more than 10 percent alcohol. The FDA has temporarily exempted homeopathic remedies from the alcohol-limit rule.

However, not all homeopathic products are exempt from the FDA rules. If a homeopathic remedy claims to cure a serious disease, such as cancer, it must be sold as a prescription drug. Only products for treating minor conditions can be sold over-the-counter.[18]

There are major differences between herbal supplements and homeopathic remedies. Herbal supplements are mainly derived from plant sources, while the active ingredients in homeopathic remedies are derived from plant, animal, and mineral sources. However, the major difference is in the amount of active ingredient present. Herbal supplements are prepared by extracting various parts of a plant, and the amount of an active ingredient in one dosage of an herbal supplement is comparable to the amount present in a single dosage of a conventional medicine (tablet, capsule, or oral liquid). In contrast, one dosage of a homeopathic remedy at 30x potency contains not even one molecule of the active ingredient. *U.S. News & World Report* has explained homeopathic dilution as follows:

> Most homeopathic remedies are diluted down to 30x, which means one drop of the active ingredient in the mother tincture was diluted with nine drops of alcohol or water, and then a drop of new solution is further diluted with 9 drops. This process continues 30 times in order to achieve 30x strength of a homeopathic remedy. It has been estimated that at this dilution, hypothetically one drop of the active ingredients is present in a container containing diluent and the size of the container is 50 times [that of] the size of the earth.[19]

Because of these extreme dilutions, toxicity and interaction with Western drugs are rarely encountered in the use of homeopathic remedies. For example, *Hypericum* (the plant also known as St. John's wort) is used in homeopathic remedies, but there is no reported therapeutic failure of any Western drug in a patient using *Hypericum*-containing homeopathy remedy. In contrast, there are many reports of reduced efficacy of Western drugs in patients taking St. John's wort herbal supplements.

The 1995 retail sales of homeopathic medicine in the United States were estimated to be $201 million, and sales were growing at a rate of 20 percent per year according to the American Association of Homeopathic Pharmacists. The number of homeopathic practitioners in the United States increased from fewer than two hundred in 1970s to approximately three thousand in 1996. The American Medical Association currently neither accepts nor rejects homeopathy.[20]

Common Homeopathic Remedies

In his early days of practicing homeopathy, Samuel Hahnemann described twenty-seven homeopathic remedies, but in his lifetime the number of remedies grew significantly due to his devoted research and that of others in this field. Today there are more than twenty-five hundred substances described in the homeopathic literature. The description of symptoms is based on the process of "proving" (the substance indicated for curing a particular illness should produce symptoms of disease in a healthy person given repeated doses of the diluted product). The first proving was performed by Hahnemann when he used cinchona bark on himself. There may be a number of remedies for a particular illness, and selection of the particular remedy is based on a detailed evaluation of the physical and mental status of the patient. A cross-reference tool used for selecting a group of remedies that correspond closely to particular symptoms is called a repertory, and the practice of using these was also introduced by Hahnemann. Modern repertories are computerized, and a homeopathic practitioner can search several databases to select one or more remedies for a particular illness. Then a thorough knowledge of the toxicological picture of the remedies, in addition to his or her own experience with them, help the practitioner to select a particular remedy for the patient.[21]

One homeopathic remedy for acute injury is *Arnica montana*, which is derived from mountain daisy. It is primarily used for the treatment of pain and bruising. However, more than one remedy is available to treat a particular condition. For example, *Aconitum napellus, Allium cepa, Arsenicum album,* belladonna, *Ferrum phosphoricum,* gelsemium, Kali bichromicum, pulsatilla, and *Rhus toxicodendron* can be used to treat symptoms of the common cold. A homeopathic practitioner, after carefully evaluating all symptoms in the patient, selects one remedy that would be most useful to treat the particular mix of these symptoms. Homeopathy relies heavily on observation and experience, and the remedy is prescribed on the totality of a person's symptoms and not just the disease.[22] For example, a homeopathic practitioner would treat a patient suffering from a cold with *Allium cepa* (onion extract) if symptoms are watering and irritation of the eyes and thin, clear nasal discharge, because these symptoms mimic those produced when a healthy person peels onions. On the other hand, a practitioner might treat another person suffering from a cold with pulsatilla (Pasque flower) when symptoms are thick, yellow nasal discharge, loss of thirst, and the desire for cool, fresh air. Although both patients are suffering from upper-respiratory-tract infection, homeopathic medicine would treat them differently.[23] Commonly used homeopathic remedies are summarized in Table 5.2. Today the ten most common diseases treated by homeopathic practitioners are asthma, depression, otitis media (middle-ear infection), hay fever, headache and migraine, neurotic disorders, other allergies, dermatitis, arthritis, and hypertension (high blood pressure).[24]

TABLE 5.2: Commonly Used Homeopathic Remedies

REMEDY	PREPARED FROM	INDICATED FOR*
Aconitum napellus	Monkshood	Fear, shock, fever, cold
Allium cepa	Onion	Itching eyes, hay fever, cold
Apis mellifica	Honeybee	Allergy, bee sting, arthritis
Arnica montana	Wolfsbane, mountain tobacco	Pain, bruising
Arsenicum album	Mineral salt (arsenic trioxide)	Cold, flu, diarrhea
Belladonna	Deadly nightshade	High fever with delirium
Bryonia alba	White bryony	Fever, cough, joint pain
Calcarea carbonica	Oyster shell	Acidity, indigestion
Calendula	Marigold	Wound healing
Ferrum phosphoricum	Mineral salt (iron salt)	Nosebleed
Gelsemium	Yellow jasmine	Fever, cold, joint pain
Hypericum	St. John's wort	Depression, skin injury, nerve pain
Kali bichromicum	Mineral salt of potassium	Respiratory-tract infection; yellow discharge from nose
Mercurius vivus	Mercury	Various chronic diseases
Natrum muriaticum	Table salt	Various chronic diseases
Nux vomica	Strychnos nux vomica tree, poison nut	Nausea, hangover
Oscillococcinum	Duck liver	Cold, flu
Phosphorus	Phosphorus	Various chronic diseases
Pulsatilla	Pasque flower, windflower	Cold, flu
Rhus toxicodendron	Poison ivy	Fever, cold, joint pain
Thuja	Northern white cedar	Warts, chronic diseases

* These are a few representative examples only. Usually a particular remedy is used to treat many different symptoms depending on the totality of symptoms in a patient.

Does Homeopathy Work? The Scientific Research

There are many stories of homeopathic treatments being successful where conventional medicine has failed. The long consultation with a homeopathic practitioner is itself therapeutic, in contrast to a visit to a physician who focuses on the illness rather than bonding with the patient. Moreover, conventional clinic settings are often ugly and sterile and can be intimidating to children. A recently published article reported on how parents of child patients experienced consultations with homeopaths and physicians. The parents felt that homeopathic consultations had a whole-person approach, while most physicians focused on the symptoms. In general, the majority of parents felt that homeopathic consultations were more beneficial.[25] In a study involving patients visiting Glasgow Homeopathic Hospital over a period of one year, the authors found that empathy is crucial in the treatment process and is strongly related to perceived changes in the main symptoms and general well-being of the patient. The length of time the practitioner spends with the patient at the initial consultation appears to be an important factor in the treatment's outcome.[26] Empathy is also emerging as a key factor in conventional medicine. Physicians who display a warm, friendly, and reassuring manner during their consultations are reported to be more effective in treating their patients.[27]

Currently, scientific methods cannot account for how homeopathic remedies work, or if they work at all. There is no known scientific basis for the like-cures-like principle. However, the greatest difficulty in explaining how homeopathic remedies work is the dilution of mother tincture. Usually it is assumed in homeopathy that the potency of a remedy becomes higher with higher dilutions. Lower potencies are used in treating physical symptoms, while higher potencies are reserved to treat physical illness with both mental and emotional components. This contrasts sharply with the molecular model of modern medicine. Homeopathy is sometimes called "ultramolecular therapy" because there may not be even one molecule of the active ingredient present in one dosage of a homeopathic remedy.

Another hypothesis of homeopathy is the idea that when a homeopathic remedy is prepared by vigorous shaking at each step the therapeutic properties of the active ingredient are transferred to water molecules (a concept sometimes referred to as "the memory of water"). Unfortunately, most scientific studies have failed to confirm this hypothesis. In one study, the author investigated fifty-seven remedies of various potencies using a very sensitive and sophisticated instrument (nuclear magnetic resonance spectrophotometer) but failed to detect any distinct signal in water molecules in any remedy that was different from the pure water molecule.[28] Most recently, it has been postulated that homeopathic remedies work through transferring information at atomic levels to water molecules in some very complex process. The "weak quantum theory" and "quantum macro-entanglement" among patients, practitioners, and remedies are new approaches to explaining how homeopathic remedies work at such high dilution levels.[29]

Although not directly related to homeopathy, one study reported that when a substance is put into distilled water and is repeatedly diluted and shaken vigorously, clusters of stable nonmelting ice crystals are formed. These crystals can be photographed using an electron microscope, which is capable of seeing very small objects almost at the molecular level. These crystals remain unchanged through subsequent dilutions. Therefore, it may be possible that water molecules in homeopathic remedies are structurally different from pure water molecules.[30]

Clinical trials evaluating the efficacy of homeopathic remedies yield conflicting results. Reports published in the journal *Homeopathy* are full of success stories, but those published in the mainstream medical journals are mixed. Some studies observed the efficacy of homeopathic remedies, while others failed to demonstrate any effect of homeopathic remedies over placebo effects.

One early clinical trial in 1835 showed that homeopathy was ineffective. This trial was very scientifically designed and is considered the birth of the modern double-blind randomized clinical trial.[31] In 2005 Shang and his colleagues published an article in the prestigious medical journal *Lancet* analyzing 110 homeopathy trials and 110 conventional medical trials. The authors concluded that biases were present in both homeopathic and conventional medical clinical trials, but there was only weak evidence for the efficacy of homeopathic remedies, while there was strong evidence of efficacy of conventional medicines. The authors further stated that the clinical effects of homeopathic remedies are placebo effects.[32] This paper raised controversy worldwide, and many professional homeopathic organizations as well as some medical researchers protested the findings. Another recently published article studied the effect of a homeopathic remedy containing *Arnica montana*, *Bryonia alba*, *Hypericum perforatum*, and *Ruta graveolens* in reducing pain following knee surgery. The authors found no effectiveness of this homeopathic remedy in reducing twenty-four-hour morphine consumption by patients.[33]

However, some clinical trials have observed the efficacy of various homeopathic remedies. Witt et al. studied a total of 3,981 patients, of which 2,851 were adults who suffered from chronic conditions—most frequently from allergic rhinitis (hay fever) or headache—and 1,130 children with atopic dermatitis (a type of eczema). The authors observed marked and sustained improvements in quality of life in patients following homeopathic treatments and concluded that homeopathy may play a beneficial role in long-term care of patients with chronic diseases.[34] Another study, this one of children between the ages of one and six, reported that over a period of twelve months, similar improvements in symptoms and quality of life were observed in children who received conventional medical treatment and those who received homeopathic treatment.[35] *Oscillococcinum*, a homeopathic remedy prepared from duck liver and heart, is effective for the treatment of influenza but cannot prevent it. *Galphimia glauca* has some efficacy in treating allergic rhinitis (hay fever).[36]

Based on detailed evaluation of sixty homeopathic clinical trials, Kleijnen and colleagues, in a paper published in the very prestigious *British Medical Journal*, concluded that they would be ready to accept that homeopathy can be efficacious if only the mechanism of action were more plausible.[37] In a study using nineteen patients, Weiser et al. compared the efficacy of a homeopathic remedy Vertigoheel (containing *Cocculus indicus, Conium maculatum, Ambra grisea,* and petroleum in a lactose base) with that of a conventional medicine (betahistine) for treating vertigo and concluded that both the homeopathic remedy and the conventional drug reduced the frequency, duration, and intensity of vertigo attacks during a six-month period. [38] Another study, by Bell et al., observed beneficial effects of individually chosen homeopathic remedies in reducing tender-point pain and improving the quality of life in patients suffering from fibromyalgia.[39]

Adverse Effects

One advantage of homeopathic treatment is its purported safety. A homeopathic practitioner matches the symptoms of the person to an effective remedy. If the match is correct, then the remedy can stimulate the body's ability to heal the illness. If the remedy choice is incorrect, usually no damage is done to the patient.[40] Homeopathic remedies have remarkably fewer side effects than conventional medicines. There are only isolated reports of adverse reactions from the use of homeopathic remedies in the medical literature. In contrast, approximately 6.7 percent of patients suffer from adverse drug reactions from conventional drug therapy and in 1994 an estimated 106,000 patients in the United States died due to adverse drug reactions.[41] In contrast, the medical literature has reported no death solely from homeopathic treatment.

Chakraborti et al. reported three cases of arsenic toxicity in patients taking arsenic-containing homeopathic remedies. All three patients took low-potency (1x) doses of various remedies, and all three showed elevated arsenic concentrations in the blood. The authors concluded that arsenic used therapeutically in homeopathic medicines can cause clinical toxicity if medications are improperly used.[42] However, in contrast to the 1x strength of the remedy described in this article, most homeopathic remedies are diluted to 30x. It is unlikely that one would encounter any serious adverse reaction from using homeopathic remedies at such a dilution. There is no known allergic reaction to homeopathic remedies because they are highly diluted. In addition, there is no known interaction of any homeopathic remedy with conventional medicine.

Conclusion

Homeopathic remedies are safe and some of them are also effective. Most homeopathic remedies come at 6c, 12c, 30c, or 30x potencies. Among complementary and alternative medicines that are taken orally, homeopathic remedies probably have the best safety records. Currently, all over-the-counter homeopathic remedies sold in the United States are oral formulations. These should be allowed to dissolve under the tongue to provide the most benefit. Although homeopathic remedies are nontoxic, it is important to select a proper remedy to treat a particular illness. It takes years of training and experience to be proficient in homeopathic practice. For treating any chronic symptoms, it is advisable that a homeopathic practitioner select your remedy rather than selecting one based on talking to friends. For children, you should consult a homeopathic practitioner before giving them any homeopathic remedy. For acute conditions such as muscle pain, you can apply arnica gel without consulting a homeopathic practitioner.

CHAPTER 6

Vitamins and Minerals

Vitamins are probably the best-selling dietary supplements in the United States, where an estimated 35 percent of the population (more than 100 million people) take multivitamin and mineral supplements. In addition, 5.2 percent of the population take vitamin B complex, and 12.7 percent take vitamin E.[1]

Vitamins are organic compounds required in very small amounts for growth and good health. Vitamins are essential for the function of certain enzymes in our body and may act as coenzymes or precursors for enzyme cofactors. In addition, certain vitamins play important roles in cell and tissue growth and cell-to-cell communication. They also provide antioxidant defense, which is vital in maintaining good health and for preventing certain diseases. Since our body cannot produce them, we must get most of our vitamins from a balanced diet. Microorganisms in our intestine commonly known as "gut flora" produce vitamin K and biotin. One form of vitamin D, however, is produced in our skin when the skin is exposed to sunlight, which contains ultraviolet rays.

Vitamins can be broadly classified into two categories: fat-soluble and water-soluble. Fat-soluble vitamins can be stored in our bodies; water-soluble vitamins cannot. Recommended daily allowances (RDAs) for adults are well established, but sick people, children, and pregnant women may require a higher intake of certain vitamins.

Minerals and trace elements are inorganic compounds that are also essential for certain vital biochemical reactions in our body. If the daily requirement is over 100 mg per day, the substance is termed a mineral. If the daily requirement is less than 100 mg per day, the substance is called a trace element.[2] Vitamins, essential minerals, and trace elements are listed in Table 6.1 on the next page.

Table 6.1: Vitamins, Essential Minerals, and Trace Elements

Classification	Individual Substance
Essential elements	Chromium, cobalt, copper, fluoride, iodide, iron, manganese, molybdenum, selenium, zinc
Fat-soluble vitamins	Vitamins A, D, E, K
Probable essential elements	Aluminum, boron, cadmium, nickel, silicon, tin
Water-soluble vitamins	Vitamins B_1 (thiamine), B_2 (riboflavin), B_3 (niacin), B_5 (pantothenic acid), B_6 (pyridoxine), B_7 (biotin), B_9 (folate), B_{12} (cyanocobalamin), C (ascorbic acid)

Vitamin A

Vitamin A, a fat-soluble vitamin, exists in two distinct forms, A_1 (retinol) and A_2 (3-dehydroretinol). Retinol, the major form of vitamin A, is found in animal liver, meat, whole milk, eggs, and some fish oil. Many breakfast cereals, fruit juices, and other foods are fortified with retinol. Our body is capable of making vitamin A from beta-carotene, a dark-colored plant pigment that is found in abundance in many fruits and vegetables such as carrots, pumpkin, sweet potatoes, cantaloupe, apricots, broccoli, spinach, and other dark-green, leafy vegetables.

Vitamin A plays many vital roles in the body, including being essential to the proper functioning of the retinas of the eyes, especially when trying to see in low light. Vitamin A helps to maintain healthy teeth, skin, and soft tissue and may protect the body against cancer. Beta-carotene, which is the precursor of vitamin A, also plays an important role as an antioxidant, protecting us from various diseases, including cancer.

The recommended daily requirement of vitamin A is 700 mcg for women (2,310 international units, or IU) and 900 mcg for men (3,000 IU). Vitamin A deficiency causes night blindness and reduces the body's capacity to fight disease. Although vitamin A deficiency is common among children in developing countries, it is rare in the United States. Daily intake of up to 3,000 mcg of vitamin A is considered safe, but excess vitamin A intake may cause toxicity, including increased risk of hip fracture and birth defects. No one—and especially not pregnant women—should consume excess vitamin A. Excess intake of vitamin A also interferes with absorption of vitamin D, causing vitamin D deficiency. Interestingly, beta-carotene, the precursor of vitamin A, is not toxic. If the body has enough vitamin A, then it does not make any from beta-carotene. Excess beta-carotene may turn your skin yellow, but that is not an adverse effect.[3]

Vitamin B Complex

Historically, it was thought that vitamin B was a single entity. In fact, there are actually eight B vitamins: B_1 (thiamine), B_2 (riboflavin), B_3 (niacin), B_5 (pantothenic acid), B_6 (pyridoxine), B_7 (biotin), B_9 (folate), and B_{12} (cyanocobalamin). Vitamin supplements containing all eight B vitamins are often referred to as vitamin B complex. Although each B vitamin has a distinct chemical structure and works independently of the others, the B vitamins often work together to support and increase the body's rate of metabolism (processing of carbohydrates, fats, and proteins for vital processes), so that we feel well and get enough energy for our activities. In particular, vitamins B_1, B_2, B_3, and B_7 participate in various aspects of energy production; vitamin B_6 participates in the metabolism of amino acids, and vitamins B_9 and B_{12} are essential for the development of red blood cells and the prevention of anemia. In addition, B vitamins play important roles in maintaining healthy skin and muscle tone as well as immune function and promoting cell growth and division—essentials for all living organisms.

Vitamin B_1 is required by all of our cells for energy metabolism. Deficiency of vitamin B_1 is often found in elderly people, as well as in alcoholics, people undergoing kidney dialysis, and individuals with chronic fatigue syndrome.[4] Vitamin B_1 deficiency causes beriberi, a disease of the nervous system. Whole wheat, peas, peanuts, fish, and meat are good sources of vitamin B_1.

Vitamin B_2 is also essential for energy metabolism. A deficiency of vitamin B_2, which may occur among alcoholics, can cause canker sores or cracks in the lips.

Niacin, vitamin B_3, is essential for the body not only for energy metabolism but also for regulating cholesterol. A niacin supplement is used for reducing cholesterol levels in the blood. Deficiency of niacin may cause pellagra, a common fatal disease, now very rare in developed countries, manifested by skin rash, diarrhea, and mental confusion.

Pantothenic acid, vitamin B_5, is essential for energy production and also to make acetylcholine (a neurotransmitter), which is necessary for healthy function of the nervous system.

If you have canker sores due to a transient (mild, short-term) deficiency of vitamin B_2, taking a vitamin B_2 supplement (there are many brands available) for two to three days will heal them. Do not take more than 30 mg a day.

Folate, vitamin B_9, is an essential supplement for pregnant women because deficiency causes neural tube defect, a serious birth defect in which the tube that forms the spinal cord and spine in the fetus does not close properly. The most common forms of neural-tube defects are spina bifida, in which lack of closure of the spinal cord and damage to the developing spine may lead to paralysis, and anencephaly, in which much of the brain does not develop. Babies with anencephaly are usually stillborn or die shortly after birth. It is better to take folate supplement even before conception to prevent neural-tube defect because every pregnant woman may be at risk. A pregnant woman needs 400 mcg a day, which is difficult to obtain from diet alone. This is the reason the FDA now requires that folate be added to most enriched breads, flour, pasta, rice, and other grain products, along with the iron and other micronutrients that have been added to these food products for many years. Although there are both genetic and environmental factors associated with the development of neural-tube defects, up to 70 percent of these defects can be prevented by maternal folic acid supplements.[5]

> *It is essential for pregnant women to take a folic acid supplement to avoid neural-tube birth defects. Your doctor will recommend which particular supplement you should take.*

The words *folate* and *folic acid* are often encountered in discussions of vitamins. Folate is the natural form of vitamin B_9. Folic acid is the form found in multivitamin complexes and in fortified foods. When we eat, folate from the food is converted into folic acid during digestion and is absorbed and used by our bodies. When folic acid is taken as a supplement, this extra step of folate conversion can be avoided and our bodies can directly absorb and use it.

Vitamin B_6 plays a role in red blood cell formation, along with vitamin B_{12} and folate. B_6 is also needed for normal reproductive function and healthy pregnancies. It has been hypothesized that folate, vitamin B_6, and vitamin B_{12} may decrease the risk for diseases and heart attack by lowering the concentration of homocysteine, an amino acid. It is known that blood homocysteine levels are elevated in people who have low blood folate, vitamin B_6, and vitamin B_{12} levels. In almost two-thirds of all patients with high homocysteine, there was low vitamin status and intake. Elevated homocysteine is associated with increased risk of cardiovascular diseases, including heart failure and stroke, and mortality from such diseases. It is also linked to increased incidence of bone fractures as well as risk of developing dementia and Alzheimer's disease.[6] The efficacy of folate, vitamin B_6, and vitamin B_{12} supplement in reducing homocysteine levels and thus the risk of heart disease has been debated. Some reports have shown benefits of such supplements in reducing the risk of heart disease, while the authors in a recent article published in the prestigious *Journal of the American Medical Association*, reporting on a study using 3,906 patients, concluded that there was no effect of receiving a supplement of folic acid, vitamin B_{12}, and vitamin B_6 on total mortality or cardiovascular events. However, therapy with folic acid/vitamin B_{12} reduced homocysteine concentration in the blood by 30 percent.[7] Folic-acid supplementation, along with vitamin B_{12} or vitamin B_6, could reduce the risk of stroke.[8]

Folate is also instrumental in preventing cancer. One study involving 88,756 women from the Nurses' Health Study reported that people who get more folic acid (more than 400 mcg per day) than an average person gets from her diet (200 mcg or less per day) or who take folic-acid supplements for more than fifteen years have a lower risk of developing colon cancer. Interestingly, no benefit from a multivitamin supplement containing folate was observed in reducing the risk of cancer in women four years after initiation of taking such supplements. There were some nonsignificant reductions in risk after ten to fourteen years of using such supplements, but after fifteen years of use, the risk of developing colon cancer was markedly reduced.[9] Folate is also useful in lowering the risk of breast cancer among postmenopausal women.[10]

Many foods are excellent sources of folate and various B vitamins. Wheat germ, whole-grain cereals, and brewer's yeast provide vitamins B_1 and B_2. These vitamins are found in beer, which contains high amounts of brewer's yeast, but they may not be present in filtered beer. These vitamins are also found in fish, meat, and milk. In addition, drinking alcohol interferes with the absorption of vitamins. Certain foods such as potatoes, bananas, lentils, peppers, liver, turkey, fish, poultry, lean meats, and molasses are good sources of various B vitamins, but vitamin B_{12} is found only in animal sources. Vegetarians and vegans are at risk of developing vitamin B_{12} deficiency. Because the stomach is required to liberate vitamin B_{12} from food, elderly people who often produce lower amounts of stomach acid may be deficient in vitamin B_{12}. Symptoms include tingling in the hands and legs, disorientation, and possible memory loss. Some Alzheimer's patients suffer from vitamin B_{12} deficiency. The fortification of food with folic acid and various vitamins has increased the percentage of adults living in the United States who have adequate levels of folate and vitamins. However, not all adults live on healthy diets, and vitamin deficiencies may occur even in healthy people. Although folate intake increased dramatically after the folic-acid fortification of food began in 1996, serum folate levels in U.S. adults have declined since then, which may be attributable to lower folic-acid intake.[11] The daily recommendations of various B vitamins are shown in Table 6.2.

TABLE 6.2: Recommended Daily Allowances (RDA) of Vitamins

VITAMIN	DEFICIENCY MAY CAUSE	RDA
Vitamin A	Night blindness	900 mcg men/700 mcg women
Vitamin B_1 (thiamine)	Beriberi	1.2 mg men/1.1 mg women
Vitamin B_2 (riboflavin)	Canker sores, eczema	1.7 mg
Vitamin B_3 (niacin)	Pellagra, skin rash, dementia	16 mg men/14 mg women
Vitamin B_5 (pantothenic acid)	Deficiency extremely rare	5 mg men/6 mg women
Vitamin B_6 (pyridoxine)	Muscle weakness	1.3 mg adults under fifty/ 1.7 mg men over fifty/ 1.5 mg women over fifty
Vitamin B_7 (biotin)	Deficiency extremely rare	30 mcg
Vitamin B_9 (folate)	Weight loss, birth defects	400 mcg
Vitamin B_{12} (cyanocobalamin)	Anemia	2.4 mcg
Vitamin C (ascorbic acid)	Scurvy, bleeding gums	90 mg men/75 mg women
Vitamin D	Rickets, poor bone/muscle strength	5–10 mcg
Vitamin E	Muscle fatigue, hair loss	15 mg
Vitamin K	Spontaneous bleeding	70–80 mcg men/60–65 mcg women

Vitamin C

The beneficial effects of vitamin C, a water-soluble vitamin, were known long before its discovery in 1932, because it was known that eating citrus fruits prevents scurvy, a fatal disease that killed many sailors between 1500 and 1800. Although many species can synthesize vitamin C, humans, primates, and a few other species cannot and must obtain it from food sources. Vitamin C plays many important roles in our bodies, including helping in many enzymatic reactions. Some of these reactions are essential for collagen formation (collagen makes cartilage and various other tissues; it is the lack of collagen synthesis due to severe vitamin C deficiency that causes scurvy), while other enzymatic reactions lead to the formation of carnitine, which transports fatty acids inside the cells to be used as fuel. In addition, vitamin C is the first line of antioxidant defense in our body and protects us from many diseases. Citrus fruits are great sources of vitamin C. Drinking a glass of orange juice every day is a very healthy practice.

Since the 1940s, numerous studies have suggested that high dosages of vitamin C may prevent or reduce the symptoms of the common cold. In 1970 Professor Linus Pauling, a two-time winner of the Nobel Prize, advocated intake of large dosages of vitamin C to prevent the common cold. His conclusion was based on a single clinical trial on schoolchildren in a skiing camp in the Swiss Alps where a significant reduction in incidences of the common cold, as well as in duration of symptoms, was observed among children who took 1 g of vitamin C supplement each day. Pauling's conclusion that vitamin C has a physiological effect on the cold is correct, although he was overly optimistic with regard to the magnitude of benefits.[12] In one study, the authors analyzed data from twenty-nine clinical trials involving 11,077 subjects and concluded that taking vitamin C at a dosage of 200 mg per day or more appears to reduce the severity and duration of colds but cannot prevent colds.[13] Another researcher analyzed data from seven clinical trials involving military personnel, three trials with students staying in crowded lodgings, and two trials involving marathon runners, and concluded that vitamin C supplements are effective in significantly reducing the incidences of the common cold and even pneumonia. This study indicates that vitamin C may be effective in reducing incidence of colds among subjects who are involved in strenuous activities and those who live in a harsh environment.[14] However, due to the failure of vitamin C to reduce incidences of the common cold among the normal population, regular megadosage of vitamin C as a prophylaxis is not justified for general use. Vitamin C in higher dosages can reduce duration of a cold and could be justified for people exposed to brief periods of severe physical exercise or cold environments.[15]

The recommended vitamin C intake in the United States is 90 mg per day, and a dosage up to 2 g per day is considered safe. However, some proponents of megavitamin intake recommended daily dosage of vitamin C as high as 4 g or more. There is no known benefit of such high dosage. In fact, excess vitamin C can have various toxic effects, including impaired absorption of iron. At this point, experts recommend intake of a regular daily dosage of vitamin C, with increased dosages for individuals suffering from a common cold or other winter illnesses in order to reduce symptoms.[16]

Vitamin D

Vitamin D is a fat-soluble vitamin that is essential for proper absorption and retention of calcium and phosphorus, which are the building blocks of our bones. Vitamin D deficiency may lead to increased risk of fractures, while vitamin D supplement, especially with calcium, may prevent them.[17] Some studies indicate that vitamin D may even prevent breast, colon, and other cancers. Postmenopausal women who take vitamin D supplement may be at a lower risk for cancer. Vitamin D deficiency also causes rickets.

The best way to prevent vitamin D deficiency is to let our bodies be exposed to the sun. Our skin, when exposed to the ultraviolet rays in sunlight, is capable of producing enough vitamin D from dehydrocholesterol, which is then stored in body fat and released during the winter months when we may experience less vitamin D production by our skin. Exposure of arms and legs for five to thirty minutes between the hours of 10:00 AM and 3:00 PM twice a week is considered sufficient to obtain enough vitamin D. Even the skin of the elderly is capable of producing enough vitamin D. In addition, most tanning beds emit 2 to 6 percent ultraviolet light and are a recommended source of vitamin D when used in moderation. People who tan more easily usually have higher levels of vitamin D than nontanners. Another important factor is the latitude where we live. In the United Kingdom, for five months of the year there is insufficient sunlight for the skin to produce enough vitamin D, and demands are made on the stores produced during the previous summer and autumn months. People who live in latitudes of 65–71 degrees north, such as the Norwegian Arctic, may not get enough sun, especially during the long winter months, to produce enough vitamin D and may have to turn to vitamin D–fortified food such as milk in order to obtain the required amount. Dark skin color may also reduce the amount of vitamin D produced by the skin because the skin pigment melanin reduces the amount of ultraviolet light that can reach the layers of the skin. African Americans with very dark skin may have their ability to produce vitamin D reduced as much as 99 percent.[18]

However, too much exposure to sunlight also has associated risks such as development of melanoma (skin cancer). Unfortunately, the high global prevalence of vitamin D insufficiency, the reemergence of rickets, and scientific evidence that low levels of circulating vitamin D in the blood may increase the risk of cancer, heart disease, and immunological disorders comprise a serious public-health challenge. Fortification of milk and other food products with vitamin D is one way to combat this problem. Even in countries where certain foods are fortified with vitamin D, the deficiency exists in certain minority populations due to vegetarian diets and a low intake of milk.[19] Animal products such as cod liver oil, fatty fish (tuna, salmon, catfish, herring, and sardines), eggs, and beef liver are major sources of vitamin D.

Vitamin E

A major role of vitamin E is to provide antioxidant defense for our bodies. Many fruits and vegetables, such as avocado, almonds, asparagus, spinach, cucumber, and nuts, as well as various vegetable oils, are rich sources of vitamin E. Although earlier studies observed beneficial effects of vitamin E supplement in preventing heart disease, more recent clinical trials failed to document any significant beneficial effect. However, a recent study showed a marked reduction in heart disease among people with type 2 diabetes who took vitamin E supplement. These patients are at higher risk of developing heart disease due to greater oxidative stress, and vitamin E may have reduced that stress in these patients.[20] The daily recommended intake of vitamin E is 15 mg.

Vitamin K

Vitamin K is instrumental in making four out of the thirteen proteins required for blood to clot, without which we would bleed to death. Vitamin K is found in many foods, including green, leafy vegetables (e.g., lettuce); broccoli; brussels sprouts; cauliflower; parsley; commonly used cooking oils; some fruits, such as avocado and kiwi; and eggs. The daily recommended intake is 120 mcg. Vitamin K also plays a role in building bones. In one study, women who got at least 110 mcg of vitamin K per day were 30 percent less likely to have a hip fracture than women who received a lower daily amount.[21]

Because vitamin K plays an important role in blood clotting, patients receiving anticoagulation therapy with warfarin should consult their doctors regarding their intake of leafy vegetables, cauliflower-type vegetables, and avocado.

Vitamin Toxicity

B vitamins, which are water-soluble, are mostly nontoxic, but vitamin C, which is also soluble in water, may cause some toxicity. Unfortunately, fat-soluble vitamins such as A, D, E, and K can cause substantial toxicity if consumed in high dosages. Because fat-soluble vitamins are stored in our body, any toxicity they cause may have long-lasting effects, so care must be taken not to consume too much of these vitamins. Fat-soluble antioxidant vitamins, if taken in larger dosages than recommended, may cause more harm than good. Miller et al. analyzed data from nineteen clinical trials involving 135,967 patients and observed that in eleven trials where high dosages of vitamin E were used (more than 400 IU a day) there was an increase in mortality from all causes. The author concluded that high dosage of vitamin E should be avoided.[22] Another recent study using data from sixty-eight clinical trials involving 232,608 subjects indicated that use of antioxidant supplements increases mortality by 5 percent. Specifically, the use of beta-carotene increased the risk of death by 7 percent, vitamin A by 16 percent, and vitamin E by 4 percent. These antioxidant vitamins, used in combination, also increased the risk of death by 16 percent. However, no adverse effect of water-soluble vitamin C was found, and the supplement selenium also was not associated with higher mortality. It is possible that these synthetic vitamins were not subjected to rigorous toxicological studies, and these results may not be applicable to natural vitamins found in foods.[23] This study was publicized by the media and generated controversy among scientists, many of whom challenged the study's design and the interpretation of its results.

Scientists of the National Cancer Institute reported that although there is no association between normal multivitamin use (once daily) and the risk of prostate cancer, there is an increased risk of advanced and fatal prostate cancer in men who take excessive multivitamin supplements (more than seven times per week). The positive association between multivitamin use and prostate cancer was strongest in men with a family history of prostate cancer or who took other supplements, including selenium, beta-carotene, and zinc.[24] See Table 6.2 on page 92 for the RDAs of various vitamins.

Mineral/Trace Elements

In addition to vitamins, minerals and trace elements are essential for sustaining life. Trace elements, or micronutrients, are defined as elements required only in minute amounts on a daily basis. In general, a balanced, healthy diet should satisfy all of our need for minerals and trace elements. Manganese, zinc, and chromium are needed in modest amounts. For physically active persons, adequate amounts of these trace elements are needed in the diet to ensure the capacity for increased energy expenditure and work performance. However, for a physically inactive person, indiscriminate use of mineral supplements can adversely affect physiological function and health.[25]

Chromium is needed to maintain stable blood-sugar levels because it controls insulin and other enzymes and helps maintain energy levels. A shortage of chromium may cause fatigue, anxiety, and glucose intolerance (high blood sugar). However, only 120 mcg a day is needed. Chromium picolinate is used as a supplement.

Copper is required for forming hemoglobin, the red pigment of blood that carries oxygen, is necessary for maintaining healthy bones, and also helps in wound healing. Copper is found in many foods, including whole grains, liver, nuts, and molasses. Taking large amounts of vitamin C and zinc may impair the absorption of copper. The intake of 1 mg of copper each day from the diet is sufficient to satisfy your body's need.

Iron is an essential element in the hemoglobin molecule and an important component of many enzymes. A deficiency of iron causes anemia. Anemia during pregnancy may increase the risk of having a premature baby or a baby with low birth weight. Therefore, both vitamin and iron supplements are essential during pregnancy. The required amount of iron is 10 mg per day in males and 18 mg for females. However, iron is toxic if taken in excess. Taking excessive iron during pregnancy may cause birth defects or spontaneous abortion. In children, doses as low as 600 mg can be fatal. Iron can be obtained through the consumption of meat, beans, nuts, fish, cereals, fruits, and vegetables.

Manganese is needed for energy, the formation of sex hormones, the production of breast milk, and the proper utilization of certain vitamins. The daily requirement is only 2 mg. Manganese is found in eggs, brown rice, leafy vegetables, and whole grains.

Zinc is required for maintaining a healthy immune system and muscle tone; the daily requirement is only 11 mg per day. Deficiency of zinc may cause fatigue, allergies, white spots under the fingernails, and skin problems, but an excess intake of zinc (1–2 g per day) may cause toxicity, including harm to the immune system. Zinc is found in fish, poultry, and meats as well as in whole grains, brewer's yeast, and eggs.

Selenium is an important trace element that protects our bodies from harmful free radicals by acting as an antioxidant. It also helps in fighting infection and producing sperm and may also have some anticancer effect. Only 55 mcg per day is needed. Selenium is found in whole grains and shellfish.

Cobalt is an integral part of vitamin B_{12} and is useful in preventing anemia. It is obtained through the consumption of a normal diet, and deficiency is unlikely.

Molybdenum, found in many food sources such as milk, lima beans, liver, and leafy vegetables, is required in a very small quantity (50 mcg), but excess consumption (over 15 mg per day) may cause toxicity.

Calcium is essential for building bones, and our daily requirement is 1,000 mg. A calcium supplement is important for most postmenopausal women, but one size does not fit all and not every postmenopausal woman needs this supplement. It is best to consult your doctor to see whether you should take a calcium and vitamin D supplement or a calcium supplement alone. Milk is a good source of calcium, and a recent study demonstrates that drinking milk for six weeks offers valuable osteoporosis prevention.[26] Also, simply drinking tea can help prevent bone loss in older women.[27]

Phosphorus is also a component of bone and plays an important role in energy processing. In the body, phosphorus is usually present as phosphate. The daily requirement is 700 mg.

In addition to these minerals, several inorganic nonmetallic elements such as fluoride, iodide, silicone, and boron are required for good health. Fluoride is essential for preventing dental cavities, and most toothpastes contain fluoride. It is also found in some drinking water and in vegetables that grow in fluoride-rich soil. Excess fluoride may stain the teeth and can be toxic.

Iodine is an essential component of thyroid hormone, and iodine deficiency may cause goiter. Salts are fortified with iodide, a form of iodine, and various seafoods are rich iodide sources, as are milk and eggs.

Silicon (silica) keeps bones, cartilage, nails, hair, and skin healthy and is found in onions, barley, rice, whole grains, and leafy vegetables.

Boron enhances the body's ability to use calcium, magnesium, and vitamin D. Dates, prunes, raisins, nuts, grapes, pears, and leafy vegetables are good sources of boron.

Do We Need Vitamin/Mineral Supplements?

Data from the 1999–2000 National Health and Nutrition Examination Survey indicate that 35 percent of Americans take multivitamin/multimineral supplements, usually a standard or senior formula, and 12–13 percent of Americans take a supplement that also contains vitamins C and E. Of the people surveyed, 10 percent take calcium supplements, 5 percent use B complex vitamins, 1.2 percent take vitamin A, 1.2 percent take vitamin B_{12}, and 1.4 percent take folic acid. Of single-mineral supplements, 2.2 percent use chromium, 1.8 percent iron, 1.1 percent selenium, and 1.1 percent zinc. Less than 1 percent of people surveyed use thiamine, riboflavin, niacin, vitamin B_6, vitamin K, beta-carotene, molybdenum, magnesium, and multimineral supplements.[28]

If you are healthy and eat a balanced diet, usually you do not need any vitamin and mineral supplements. However, most Americans do not eat a balanced, healthy diet, and some healthy individuals do suffer from deficiency of certain vitamins. Vegetarians often suffer from vitamin B_{12} deficiency, and in one study, 60 percent of vegetarians had subclinical stage 3 vitamin B_{12} deficiency (stage 4 deficiency produces clinically recognized symptoms).[29] On the other hand, not eating enough fruits and vegetables every day and eating too much meat may produce deficiencies of other vitamins and minerals.

> *Taking one multivitamin/mineral supplement each day is a good idea to prevent any potential vitamin or mineral deficiency in a healthy individual. Do not take more than one multivitamin/mineral supplement per day unless your doctor recommends a higher intake.*

When selecting a supplement, read labels carefully. It is recommended that you take a product with vitamins in amounts comparable to RDA values or slightly above them. The amount of each vitamin/mineral should be significantly below the tolerable upper intake level of each vitamin/mineral (see Table 6.3 on the next page). For healthy individuals there is no reported advantage to taking megavitamin supplements, and excess vitamin intake may cause more harm than good. In general there is no known scientific advantage to taking organic vitamins over taking a general brand-name multivitamin supplement.

TABLE 6.3: Tolerable Upper Intake Level of Certain Vitamins and Supplements[30]

VITAMIN/MINERAL	TOLERABLE UPPER INTAKE LEVEL
Vitamin A	2,000 mcg
Vitamin B$_3$ (niacin)	35 mg
Vitamin B$_6$ (pyridoxine)	100 mg
Vitamin B$_9$ (folate)	1,000 mcg
Vitamin C	2,000 mg
Vitamin E	1,000 mg
Calcium	2,500 mg
Copper	10 mg
Iron	45 mg
Phosphorus	3,500 mg
Zinc	40 mg

One study reports that a large number of American children and adolescents use vitamin and mineral supplements that may not be medically required.[31] In another study, the authors reported that vitamin/mineral supplement use among toddlers was associated with being a firstborn child and a picky eater. The authors concluded that generally healthy infants and toddlers can obtain recommended levels of vitamins and minerals through diet alone, and caregivers should be encouraged to use food rather than supplements as the primary source of nutrition in children. Vitamin and mineral supplements can help infants and toddlers with special nutrient needs, but caution should be exercised to avoid vitamin overdoses, especially for vitamin A, zinc, and folate.[32] However, pregnant women require daily vitamin and mineral supplements, especially folate and iron, and it is always wise to strictly follow the recommendation of your doctor in taking such supplements, because taking more vitamins than recommended may potentially harm you. Like pregnant women, elderly people are a population that has to be vigilant about preventing vitamin deficiency. Regardless of your situation, remember that it is best to follow the recommendation of your doctor when it comes to taking multivitamin/mineral supplements.

Conclusion

Despite extensive research, currently there is no documented proof that taking multivitamin and mineral supplements will prevent disease or increase longevity.

Huang et al. concluded that at this point, evidence is insufficient to prove the presence or absence of benefits from use of multivitamin and mineral supplements to prevent cancer and chronic diseases.[33] Millions of postmenopausal women use multivitamins, often believing that supplements prevent chronic diseases such as cancer and cardiovascular diseases. Neuhouser et al., studying 161,808 participants from the Women's Health Initiative clinical trials or observational studies involving 93,676 women, concluded that after a median follow-up of eight years there was no convincing evidence that multivitamin supplements prevent cancer, cardiovascular disease, or total mortality in postmenopausal women.[34]

Therefore, it is wise not to spend too much money on producing expensive urine (excess water-soluble vitamins are excreted in the urine). Eating a healthy diet that includes meats, poultry, vegetables, grains, and fruits each day is the best way to fulfill our daily requirements of vitamins and minerals. Try to avoid eating fast food. Daily exercise is helpful in maintaining good health. If you are healthy, you can take one multivitamin/mineral supplement per day, but please do not take vitamins in excess unless your doctor recommends such use, because excess multivitamin/mineral intake may cause harm.

CHAPTER 7

Moderately Toxic Herbal Remedies That May Cause Organ Damage

Several herbal remedies are known to cause organ damage. Usually, injuries to organs, especially the liver and kidneys, appear to result from taking high doses of these remedies for a few months or more, but some of these remedies are more toxic and may cause organ damage within a few weeks or even days. Several drugs are also known to cause liver damage, and if any herbal supplement such as kava is taken at the same time as one of these drugs, the possibility of liver damage may increase. Table 7.1 lists common drugs that may cause liver damage; Table 7.2 lists common drugs that may cause kidney damage. Because the pharmacology and toxicology of these drugs are well documented, your doctor is aware of such toxicity and will monitor your blood levels of liver enzymes to check your liver function. Moreover, over-the-counter medications such as aspirin, acetaminophen, and other pain relievers can cause both liver and kidney damage if taken for a long period of time.

TABLE 7.1: Some Common Drugs That May Cause Liver Damage

CLASS OF MEDICATION	DRUG
Analgesic	Aspirin, acetaminophen (Tylenol), diclofenac, indomethacin
Antibiotic	Tetracycline, erythromycin, isoniazid
Antigout	Allopurinol
Anticonvulsant	Phenytoin, valproic acid
Cardioactive	Amiodarone, quinidine
Cholesterol-lowering	Niacin, statins

TABLE 7.2: Some Common Drugs That May Cause Kidney Damage

CLASS OF MEDICATION	DRUG
Analgesic	Acetaminophen (Tylenol), aspirin, other nonsteroidal anti-inflammatory drugs, such as ibuprofen, naproxen, etc.
Antibiotic	Tetracycline, vancomycin, tobramycin, amikacin, gentamicin, kanamycin, cephalosporin and quinolone antibiotics, sulfonamide antibiotics
Anticancer	Methotrexate
Anticonvulsant	Carbamazepine, phenytoin
Antigout	Allopurinol
Antiviral	Foscarnet, indinavir
Cardioactive	Quinidine
Immuno-suppressants	Cyclosporine, tacrolimus

Unfortunately, many patients do not tell their doctors that they are using herbal supplements, and sometimes an herbal supplement will even increase the toxicity of prescription medications. Although liver and kidney damage from herbal remedies usually occurs after at least one month of continued use, certain herbal remedies are more toxic and may cause organ damage within a few weeks or days after use.

Blood Tests to Check Liver Function

Several markers of liver injury can be tested in blood to determine the health of your liver. Alanine transaminase and aspartate transaminase (AST) are found inside the liver cells (hepatocytes), and small amounts of these enzymes can be detected in the serum of healthy individuals. However, in the case of liver injury, such as hepatitis, the activity of these enzymes may be increased five- to tenfold. Bilirubin, a breakdown product of hemoglobin in the blood, is cleared by the liver. In the case of liver injury, the bilirubin concentration in blood can become significantly elevated. Alkaline phosphatase (ALP), another enzyme found in the cell lining of the liver's biliary duct, is also elevated. The enzyme gamma-glutamyl transpeptidase (GGTP) is also a marker of liver injury and is elevated in people who drink alcohol. In addition, the liver synthesizes albumin and many other proteins. Therefore, albumin concentration may be lower in persons with significant liver damage. Normal values for these markers for liver disease are presented in

Table 7.3. Prothrombin time, a measurement of the coagulation capacity of blood, may also be altered due to liver injury.

TABLE 7.3: Normal Values for Liver-Function Tests

BLOOD COMPONENT MEASURED	NORMAL VALUE
Alanine transaminase (ALT)	5–40 units/liter (U/L)
Albumin	3.5–4.5 gm/dL
Alkaline phosphatase (ALP)	30–120 U/L
Aspartate transaminase (AST)	10–40 U/L
Bilirubin	0.2–1.5 mg/100 mL (mg/dL)
Gamma-glutamyl transpeptidase (GGT)	0–51 U/L
Total protein	6–8 gm/dL

Herbal Supplements That Cause Liver Damage

The most widely cited herbal supplement that causes liver damage is kava. There has been a significant amount of media coverage about its dangers. In 2002, ABC News, CNN Health News, and *USA Today* all warned people about liver toxicity resulting from kava consumption, following an FDA consumer advisory regarding safety risk. Chaparral, black cohosh, germander, LipoKinetix, mistletoe, pennyroyal oil, and several Chinese medicines can cause significant liver damage, and consumers should be aware of the dangers associated with these herbal supplements.

The largest documented number of cases of liver injury due to use of herbal supplements came from the Japanese Health Ministry, which cited several Asian herbal weight-loss products that caused serious toxicity, mainly in women aged twenty-three to sixty-three.[1] Two Japanese herbal weight-loss products, Chaso and Onshido, contain N-nitroso-fenfluramine, which is toxic to the liver. Although this compound is structurally similar to fenfluramine, a weight-loss product withdrawn from the market due to cardiac toxicity, fenfluramine has no known liver toxicity. Lists of the herbal supplements and traditional Chinese medicines that may cause liver toxicity are given below:

Herbal Supplements That May Cause Liver Damage

- black cohosh
- comfrey
- chaparral
- germander

- green-tea extract
- LipoKinetix
- noni juice
- kava
- mistletoe
- pennyroyal

Traditional Chinese Medicines That May Cause Liver Damage

- Chaso
- Jin Bu Huan
- Onshido
- Sho-Saiko-To
- Dai-Saiko-To
- Ma Huang
- Shen Min
- Shou Wu Pian

Asian Weight-Loss Products and Other Asian Supplements

The most dangerous Asian weight-loss product is Ma Huang, which contains ephedra alkaloids. Ma Huang may cause severe cardiac toxicity, hepatic toxicity, and even death. (Please see Chapter 8 for a more detailed discussion on Ma Huang.)

As mentioned, the weight-loss products Chaso or Onshido, which contain N-nitroso-fenfluramine, are toxic to the liver and should be avoided at all costs because death has been reported from their use. Moreover, genetic factors may play an important role in the toxicity of these products. Other Asian herbal supplements containing multiple herbs and Dai-Saiko-To or Sho-Saiko-To (also known as Kampo medicines) are known to cause liver injuries. Jin Bu Huan, which is used as a sedative analgesic, is also known to cause liver damage. Acute hepatitis has been reported in healthy individuals who used these herbal supplements. Shou Wu Pian, a proprietary Chinese medicine used for treating dizziness, back pain, and constipation, may also cause hepatitis. Shen Min, another Chinese medicine, has also been associated with drug-induced hepatitis.[2]

Black Cohosh

Black cohosh is primarily used for alleviating symptoms of menopause and sometimes for weight loss. There are several reports of liver toxicity from using black cohosh, including two persons who required liver transplants. In most cases, high serum bilirubin and liver enzymes are observed in patients after they start taking black cohosh.[3]

In one report, a fifty-year-old woman started taking black cohosh for relief of postmenopausal symptoms. She later developed fatigue and abdominal pain and was diagnosed with liver disease due to use of black cohosh. After she stopped taking black cohosh, she recovered.[4]

CASE STUDY

Recently, regulatory agencies in Australia, Canada, and the European Union have released statements regarding the potential association between use of black cohosh and liver toxicity. The Dietary Supplements Information Expert Committee of the United States Pharmacopeia determined that products containing black cohosh should have warning labels.

Chaparral

Chaparral is a plant found in the southwestern United States and northern Mexico. Its leaves are used as an herbal supplement for treating a wide variety of symptoms from cold sores to muscle pain. It is also used as an antioxidant, anti-HIV, and anticancer product. Chaparral can be taken as dried extract in capsule or tablet form. Leaves, stems, and bark are available in bulk for brewing tea. The active ingredient of chaparral is nordihydroguaiaretic acid (NDGA), which has anti-inflammatory and antioxidant properties. However, this product can cause severe toxicity to the liver. Several cases of chaparral-associated hepatitis have been reported. In one report, a forty-five-year-old woman took chaparral (160 mg/day) for ten weeks before going to the hospital with jaundice, anorexia, fatigue, nausea, and vomiting. Liver enzymes and other liver-function tests showed abnormally high values indicating severe liver injury. Normal liver enzyme ALT values in blood are up to 40 U/L; in this patient, the value was elevated to 1,611 U/L. The diagnosis was chaparral-induced cholestatic hepatitis.[5]

Sheikh et al. reviewed eighteen cases of illness from using chaparral and found thirteen cases of liver toxicity. These patients came to clinics with significantly elevated liver enzymes and other liver markers in their blood specimens, usually three to fifty-two weeks after using chaparral. After discontinuing the use of chaparral, the liver enzyme levels in the blood returned to normal values. However, chaparral-induced liver injury may be irreversible and may cause liver failure requiring transplant.[6]

> **The FDA has warned the public about the dangers of consuming chaparral.**

Comfrey

The leaves and roots of comfrey, a hardy perennial plant, are traditionally used for treating arthritis and gout, healing wounds, and repairing broken bones. It is also believed that comfrey can heal psoriasis. There is no scientific evidence to support those claims, and comfrey can cause liver injury. It contains chemicals known as pyrrolizidine alkaloids, which are known hepatotoxins (substances that are poisonous to the liver). Russian comfrey is even more toxic than comfrey found in Europe and Asia because it contains more potent hepatotoxins. Endemic outbreaks in Jamaica, India, and Afghanistan have been reported due to use of contaminated cereals containing comfrey and the use of comfrey tea. In Jamaica, toxicity was due to drinking "bush tea" as a folk medicine. It has been documented that pyrrolizidine alkaloids and their oxides are transformed into more potent hepatotoxins by the liver enzymes that metabolize drugs. The liver disease caused by comfrey is called veno-occlusive disease, which may lead to cirrhosis and eventually liver failure. Use of comfrey is banned in Germany and Canada.[7]

Germander

Germander is an aromatic plant in the mint family, and germander tea, made from the aerial parts of the plant, has been in use for many centuries. Blossoms of germander are used as a folk medicine to treat dyspepsia, diabetes, and gout. Germander has also been used for weight loss and as a general tonic. Although considered safe in the past, germander was banned by the French authorities in 1992 due to twenty-six cases of liver toxicity. The toxicity is manifested by significant increases in liver enzymes and other markers of liver injury in blood within two months of use of a germander product. Because this herb is also used for weight loss, many women were victims of this product.[8]

> **CASE STUDY**
>
> A fifty-five-year-old woman taking 1,600 mg per day of germander became jaundiced after six months. Her bilirubin was 13.9 mg/dL (normal value is up to 1.5 mg/dL), and her liver enzyme ALT was elevated to 1,500 U/L (normal ALT value is up to 40 U/L). A liver biopsy suggested drug-induced hepatitis. Germander therapy was discontinued and the hepatitis resolved in two months.

> **CASE STUDY**
>
> A forty-five-year-old woman who had taken germander (260 mg/day) for weight loss also showed high bilirubin and liver enzymes in her blood. After she discontinued use of germander, her condition improved. After four months, she felt much better and started taking germander again, and one week later she again developed liver toxicity.

Generally, the toxic effects of germander start within nine weeks of use and are manifested by jaundice (high bilirubin in blood) and elevated levels of the liver enzymes ALT and AST. After the discontinuation of germander, recovery may take six weeks to six months. The liver toxicity is related to diterpenoid compounds, which are activated and become more potent liver toxins after metabolism by the liver enzymes.[9]

Green-Tea Extract

Green tea originated in China and is prepared solely from leaves of *Camellia sinensis*. It has long been claimed to reduce risks of cancer and heart disease. The extract of green tea is also used as an herbal weight-loss product.

CASE STUDY A thirty-seven-year-old woman developed abdominal pain after using TRA (The Right Approach) Complex, a dietary supplement containing green-tea extract. The liver enzymes in her blood were elevated to more than forty times the normal values, and her liver injury was probably related to the use of green-tea extract. After discontinuation of the supplement, her liver-function tests improved over the next six weeks. But one year later, she presented with similar symptoms and admitted to using green-tea extract again a month before developing these symptoms. Once she discontinued use of the extract, the disease resolved in six months.

Two cases of acute liver failure have also been reported in the medical literature due to use of green-tea extract. One patient received a liver transplant. The mechanism of liver toxicity from consumption of green-tea extract is unclear.[10]

Kava

Kava, prepared from a South Pacific plant (*Piper methysticum*), is an herbal sedative with antianxiety effects. There are seventy-two species of the kava plant, which differ in appearance as well as chemical composition. Native South Pacific Islanders prepared kava drinks by mixing the fresh or dried root with cold water or coconut milk. Kava is available from a variety of manufacturers. Its active ingredients are called kava lactones.[11]

Despite the toxicity of kava, early scientific research indicated that its efficacy in treating anxiety disorders was comparable to that of some antidepressants and tranquilizers.[12] Chronic ingestion of kava may cause temporary yellowing of the skin, hair, and nails.

A seventy-year-old man who took kava products for anxiety for two to three weeks experienced itching several hours after exposure to the sun and developed plaques on his face, chest, and back. A similar case involved a fifty-two-year-old woman who noticed papules and plaques on her face, arms, back, and chest after taking kava products for three weeks. In both cases, biopsies revealed lymphocytic infiltration of the dermis with destruction of the sebaceous glands of the skin.[13]

Although liver damage is the most widely documented toxicity of kava, it has additive effects when taken in combination with central nervous system depressants. A patient who was taking alprazolam (Xanax), cimetidine, and terazosin became lethargic and disoriented after ingesting kava and fell into coma.[14]

Interestingly, before 1998 kava extracts were considered a safe alternative to drug therapy for treating anxiety disorders. Until that time, a number of published scientific reviews considered kava both safe and effective. Nevertheless, in 2002 the FDA released an advisory on the use of kava extract, and in 2003 kava was banned in the entire European Union and Canada. Prolonged consumption of kava has been associated with increased concentrations of gamma-glutamyl transferase (GGT; same as gamma-glutamyl transpeptidase) in blood, suggesting toxicity to the liver.

A fifty-year-old man took three to four kava capsules daily for two months (the maximum recommended dose is three capsules). Liver-function tests showed a sixty- to seventyfold increase in AST and ALT. The blood test was negative for hepatitis and HIV, indicating that the liver damage was due to the use of kava. This patient eventually received a liver transplant.[15]

One report cited eleven cases of hepatic failure requiring liver transplant and four cases of fatal incidences due to the use of kava.[16] There are twenty-four documented cases of severe liver damage in Germany due to the use of kava, including three patients requiring transplant and one death. The person who died from using kava consumed a standardized extract containing 30–70 percent kava lactones.[17]

The dangers of using kava extracts are well recognized in the medical community. However, for two thousand years, native inhabitants of the Pacific Islands (Micronesia, the Marshall Islands, Palau, and the Northern Marianas) have used kava without experiencing serious toxicity. Interestingly, many drugs used for treating anxiety and depression may also cause liver toxicity. It is believed that kava lactones, which are metabolized by the liver, are responsible for kava's toxicity. A family of liver enzymes known as cytochrome P-450 mixed function oxidase is responsible for the metabolism of kava. When a high amount of kava is ingested, this detoxification pathway is saturated, causing toxicity. Glutathione, a tripeptide (contains three amino acids) and a powerful antioxidant, plays a role in detoxification of kava lactones by the liver. With excess kava lactone in the blood, the glutathione supply in the liver may be exhausted, increasing toxicity from kava. Interestingly, acetaminophen (Tylenol) toxicity due to overdose also occurs through depletion of glutathione in the liver.

Traditionally, Pacific Islanders prepared kava drinks by steeping kava roots in water or coconut milk, or in a combination of the two. Such processes extract only a small amount of kava lactone, along with water-soluble glutathione, also found in kava roots. This glutathione protects the liver from kava toxicity. The commercial kava preparations found in health-food stores use either ethanol (alcohol) or acetone for extraction, or they use a mixture of 25 percent ethanol and 75 percent water. One published report demonstrated that the use of the traditional extract method with water resulted in the presence of only 3 percent kava lactone after drying. The authors further concluded that if a mixture of 25 percent ethanol and 75 percent water is used as an extraction solvent, 25 percent kava lactones are present in the extract. Dried extract prepared by using 100 percent ethanol contained 100 percent of kava lactones. Glutathione is insoluble in ethanol and is absent in a kava preparation if 100 percent ethanol is used for extraction. However, some glutathione may be present if a lower amount of alcohol (less than 50 percent) is used for extraction. The toxicity from the use of kava extract may be due to much-higher amounts of kava lactones being present in the commercial preparations available in health-food stores.[18]

My recommendation is not to use kava under any circumstances, even for a few weeks, just to be on the safe side.

LipoKinetix

LipoKinetix has been promoted for weight loss on the basis of the claim that it increases metabolism and can serve as an alternative to exercise. This product contains phenylpropanolamine (which is banned by the FDA in all over-the-counter cold medications), caffeine, yohimbe, diiodothyronine, and sodium usniate. In 2002, seven patients who were using LipoKinetix developed acute hepatitis.[19] The sodium usniate found in LipoKinetics is derived from usnic acid, which in turn is derived from lichen. Usnic acid has antibacterial properties and is used in skin cream and mouthwash. Liver toxicity due to its use has been documented in the medical literature. Moreover, usnic acid is present in kombucha tea (also known as Manchurian mushroom or Manchurian fungus tea), which is prepared by brewing kombucha mushrooms in sweet black tea. Acute liver damage due to drinking this tea has been reported. There may be inherent susceptivity to usnic acid toxicity due to genetic predisposition. In addition, LipoKinetix also contains the ephedra alkaloid phenylpropanolamine, which may also contribute to its hepatotoxicity.[20] The FDA has warned consumers not to take LipoKinetix (http://www.fda.gov/medwatch). Herbalife, another product promoted for weight reduction, may also cause liver injury.[21]

Mistletoe

Mistletoe is a parasitic evergreen plant that lives on trees such as oak, elm, fir, pine, and apple. It has a yellowish flower, green leaves, and waxy poisonous berries. Aside from being known as the plant people kiss beneath during the Christmas season, mistletoe was used in folk medicine as a digestive aid, heart tonic, and sedative. It was also used in treating arthritis, hysteria and other mental disturbances, cancer, and hepatitis. The mistletoe found in herbal remedies usually comes from the leaves.

> A forty-nine-year-old woman developed nausea, general malaise, and abdominal pain after using mistletoe, and liver damage caused by mistletoe was diagnosed as a result. She recovered, and two years later she developed similar symptoms after using mistletoe again. The authors concluded that mistletoe causes hepatitis.[22]

CASE STUDY

However, there are only very few reports in the medical literature of liver problems following the use of mistletoe.

Pennyroyal Oil

Oil of pennyroyal, a mint with a strong fragrance, is used in aromatherapy or as a bath additive. It is used in folk medicine for inducing abortions. Pennyroyal oil contains several components, including pulegone, a liver toxin. Pulegone is metabolized by the liver into a more toxic compound, methofuran, and is known to deplete glutathione in the liver. The toxicity is similar to that induced by an overdose of acetaminophen (Tylenol). Therefore, pennyroyal oil should never be ingested. Pennyroyal tea is also toxic and causes both hepatic and neurological damage. There are reports of an infant dying after ingesting pennyroyal tea and of another infant developing severe liver disease. There have also been reports of severe toxicity from pennyroyal oil in adults. One woman who used pennyroyal oil for inducing an abortion developed multi-organ failure and died. Important to note, N-acetylcysteine, which is used to treat acetaminophen toxicity, is also useful in treating toxicity due to ingestion of pennyroyal oil.[23] In other published papers, researchers reviewed eighteen cases of pennyroyal toxicity and concluded that even ingestion of as little as 10 mL may cause severe toxicity. One of two patients studied in detail died from ingestion of pennyroyal oil.[24] There are occasional reports of skin problems (contact dermatitis) following use of pennyroyal oil.

> *Pennyroyal oil should not be used in aromatherapy or in bath therapy because of occasional reports of skin problems associated with such use (dermatitis). It can cause severe liver disease if ingested.*

Herbal Supplements That May Cause Kidney Damage

In 1993 rapidly progressing kidney damage was reported in a group of young women who were taking pills containing Chinese herbs while attending a weight-loss clinic in Belgium. It was discovered that one prescription Chinese herb had been replaced by another Chinese herb containing aristolochic acid, a known toxin to the kidneys.[25] Later there were many reports of kidney damage due to the use of herbal supplements contaminated with aristolochic acid. The National Kidney Foundation stated that wormwood plant, sassafras, the Chinese herbal product Tung Shueh, and horse chestnut may be toxic to the kidneys. In addition, people suffering from chronic renal disease should not take alfalfa, aloe, bayberry, blue cohosh, broom, buckthorn, capsicum, cascara, coltsfoot, dandelion, ginger, ginseng, horsetail, licorice, nettle, noni juice, rhubarb, senna, vervain, or yerba maté. According to the foundation, herbals such as chaparral, comfrey, ephedra (Ma Huang), lobelia, mandrake, pennyroyal, pokeroot, sassafras, senna, and yo-himbe are unsafe and should be avoided (http://www.kidney.org/atoz/atozItem .cfm?id=123).

There are several herbal supplements that are known to cause blood in the urine (hematuria) and loss of protein in the urine (proteinuria). Examples are aloe-leaf juice, kava, and saffron. Many other herbs, such as calamus, chaparral, horse-chestnut seed, and wormwood oil, may cause kidney toxicity.[26] In addition, several herbs have diuretic effects (removing water and salt from the body) and may cause irritation to cells of the kidney (renal epithelial cells). These herbs, such as asparagus root, lovage root, parsley, watercress, and white sandalwood, should be avoided if you have any kidney problem.[27] The following herbs may cause kidney damage:

- aloe juice
- chaparral
- horse chestnut
- juniper berry
- parsley
- wormwood

- calamus
- Chinese herbs containing aristolochic acid
- horse-chestnut seed
- kava
- sassafras
- wormwood oil

Many other herbs are contraindicated if you have renal disease (see above).

Herbal Supplements Toxic to the Heart and Miscellaneous Other Toxicities

Various problems such as hypertension, electrolyte imbalance (change of sodium, potassium, and other salts in the blood), chest pain, cardiac arrhythmia, and even death due to heart failure may result from taking herbal supplements. Herbal remedies that have been implicated repeatedly in heart-related problems are aco-nite, ephedra-containing alkaloids, and licorice.[28]

Aconite is derived from the perennial plant *Aconitum* (monkshood) and is traditionally used for treating many illnesses (rheumatism, neurological prob-lems), reducing pain, and detoxification. It is also used as an active ingredient in homeopathic remedies. In homeopathic remedies it is used in extremely small amounts; therefore, toxicity is unlikely. However, severe toxicity and even death may result from using nonhomeopathic herbal supplements containing aconite. Aconite is a very toxic plant alkaloid that is well known for causing arrhythmias and even death. It is also very toxic to the nervous system. The lethal dose of aconite in humans is 2–6 mg.[29] Accidental aconite poisoning causing the death of a twenty-five-year-old man has been reported. The concentration of aconite in his blood was only 3.6 ng/mL (3.6 nanograms; one billionth of a g), an extremely low concentration.[30]

Ephedra-containing alkaloids are associated with more than one hundred reported deaths and are discussed in detail in Chapter 8. Several Chinese medicines such as Chan Su and herbal supplements containing cardiac glycosides and oleander cause heart failure and death. These herbs are also discussed in more detail in Chapter 8.

Licorice is prepared from the root of *Glycyrrhiza glabra*. Because of its sweet taste, it is used in various candies. It is also used as a cough suppressant, as a laxative, and in treating ulcers. However, licorice contains glycyrrhizinic acid, which affects the endocrine system and may also raise blood pressure. Individuals taking blood-pressure medications should not use licorice. For people in good health, taking excessive licorice may cause hypertension or loss of potassium (hypokalemia) and other electrolyte imbalances and may cause a medical emergency. Licorice should not be used by anyone taking digoxin, because licorice-induced electrolyte imbalance may cause severe digoxin toxicity, especially in the elderly. An eighty-four-year-old man who was taking digoxin experienced severe toxicity from using licorice and required hospitalization.[31]

Kelp is a kind of seaweed and contains a very high amount of iodine. Because salts we eat contain iodine, we do not need iodine supplement for our health. Eating kelp, which is indicated for hypothyroidism, may be problematic because excess iodine will cause thyroid malfunction, especially in people taking a thyroxine supplement. Taking kelp regularly increases blood concentration of thyroid-stimulating hormone (TSH). A seventy-two-year-old woman with a normal thyroid gland developed hyperthyroidism after ingesting kelp tablets. The thyroid functions returned to normal six months after discontinuation of kelp.[32] In another case report a thirty-two-year-old woman with goiter presented to the hospital with symptoms of hyperthyroidism; her problem developed four weeks after taking kelp-containing herbal tea following the recommendation of a Chinese herbal practitioner.[33] Taking iodine-containing medication such as amiodarone can also cause thyroid problems. Herbs that may cause heart problems and other problems are listed in Table 7.4.

TABLE 7.4: Herbs Causing Heart Problems and Miscellaneous Other Problems

PROBLEM	ASSOCIATED HERB
Herbs causing digoxin-like toxicity	Chan Su, oleander
Electrolyte imbalance	Aloe, buckthorn bark and berry, licorice, rhubarb root, senna leaf
Hypertension	Ephedra, Indian snakeroot, licorice, khat
Hyperthyroid	Iodine
Various heart problems	Aconite, ephedra, licorice

Conclusion

There are several herbal supplements available today that are harmful. The severity of organ damage from these herbal supplements depends on the dosage and duration of use. Taking a higher dosage for a long period is associated with more severe symptoms of organ damage. In addition, any underlying illness may affect the toxicity of an herbal supplement. It is best to talk to your health-care provider about whether or not you should take any herbal supplement at all. And always find out which ones are safe and beneficial before beginning use.

CHAPTER 8

Severely Toxic Herbal Remedies That May Even Cause Death

People turn to herbal supplements in order to avoid the toxicities and drug interactions of Western medications. Although many herbal supplements are fairly benign in the sense that they do not cause any serious adverse effects, some natural supplements are not safe at all. The May 2005 issue of *Consumer Reports* listed several cases where consuming "natural" dietary supplements causes serious side effects.[1] In general, an herbal supplement can be considered safe (see Chapter 2), moderately toxic causing organ damage, or severely toxic (supplements in this category may even cause death). Although the division between safe herbs and toxic herbs (moderately toxic and severely toxic) is clear cut, the difference between moderately toxic herbs and severely toxic herbs is not so clear, and there is an overlapping grey area. Therefore, it is possible that a moderately toxic herb could cause severe toxicity in certain individuals. Why certain moderately toxic herbs may cause severe toxicity and even death to certain individuals is poorly understood, but it may be due to differences in their genetic makeup. A detailed discussion of how genetic variations between people lead to different ways of responding to the toxicity of an herbal supplement is beyond the scope of the book. However, certain herbal supplements discussed in Chapter 7 are also briefly discussed in this chapter to emphasize the fact that such herbs, although considered to be moderately toxic, may cause severe toxicity and even fatality to some individuals. Therefore, it is wise to avoid all herbs discussed in this chapter.

CASE STUDY A twenty-one-year-old woman took Xenadrine EFX "thermogenic" diet pills to increase her energy before final exams. These pills contained bitter orange but had no ephedra-containing alkaloids, and she considered the product to be safe. Unfortunately, three weeks after taking them, she suffered from a seizure. After discontinuing the diet pills she did not have any further problems.

A fifty-nine-year-old woman went to an acupuncturist in 1992 for relief of back pain and received a selection of Chinese herbal medicines. In 1994 she developed serious kidney failure, and in 1996 she underwent a kidney transplant. Some of her Chinese herbal remedies contained aristolochic acid, a known toxin to the kidneys. The distributor of the herbal medicine said that the Chinese supplier substituted aristolochia for another herb without his knowledge.

CASE STUDY

Chinese dietary supplements contaminated with aristolochic acid have caused many cases of severe toxicity (see Chapter 7 for more details).

Fortunately, relatively small numbers of dietary supplements are toxic, but some are so toxic that they can even cause death. These herbal remedies should be avoided at all cost. In Chapter 7, herbal remedies that may cause organ damage are discussed. Some of these supplements can be considered borderline toxic. Licorice, for example, has caused adverse reactions only after heavy consumption or in a select group of people who have high blood pressure. St. John's wort is a safe and effective herbal antidepressant unless you are taking prescription drugs or if you commonly sunbathe. (Unfortunately, St. John's wort can reduce the efficacy of many drugs; see Chapter 9 for a detailed discussion of this phenomenon.)

Herbal Supplements That Are Severely Toxic

Several reports in the medical literature have reported death due to the use of an herbal supplement or an herbal tea. A number of such reports deal with Chinese medicines such as aconite-containing herbal products, products contaminated with aristolochic acid, or Chan Su. However, death has also been associated with drinking oleander tea and with taking kava supplement or other herbal products such as germander and chaparral. The most notorious herbal supplements causing multiple deaths are probably ephedra-containing herbal weight-loss products such as Ma Huang. See Table 8.1 on the next page for a list of herbs that may cause death. Readers should avoid these herbs at all costs.

TABLE 8.1: Herbal Supplements Associated with Reports of Death

HERBAL SUPPLEMENT	CAUSE OF DEATH
Aconite-containing Chinese herbs/monkshood plant	Cardiac shock/failure
Chan Su and other bufalin-containing Asian medicines	Cardiac failure
Chinese medicine containing methyl salicylate/oil of wintergreen	Metabolic acidosis
Comfrey	Liver failure
Ephedra-containing herbs	Cardiac failure
Germander	Liver failure
Kava	Liver failure
Pennyroyal oil	Liver failure
Oleander tea	Cardiac failure
Thunder-god vine	Cardiac shock/damage

Aconite

Aconite, a flowering perennial native to China and Europe, is commonly known as monkshood. Recognized as a poison for centuries, aconite is nonetheless used in a few Chinese herbal formulas and homeopathic remedies. In Chinese medicine, a small amount of aconite extract from leaves, flowers, and roots is used to treat pain due to arthritis, gout, cancer, inflammation, migraine headache, and sciatica. Because aconite is very toxic, its use can cause irregular heartbeat, heart block (a disease in the electrical system of the heart), heart failure, and death. Aconite is even dangerous in the form of cream for topical application because it can be absorbed through the skin. Merely touching this plant may cause an allergic reaction in allergy-prone individuals.

The Chinese medicines Chuan Wu and Cao Wu are prepared from roots of various species of aconite plants and are believed to have anti-inflammatory, analgesic, and cardiotonic effects. These products contain highly toxic compounds such as aconitine, mesaconitine, and hypaconitine. Death may occur as a result of ventricular arrhythmia (very abnormal heart rhythm), usually with twenty-four hours of ingestion of herbal supplements. There is no antidote to treat aconite poisoning, only supportive therapy to sustain life. In one report, three patients who consumed an aconite-containing herbal remedy died from very abnormal heart rhythm.[2] Another patient was very ill ninety minutes after taking an aconite-containing Chinese herbal preparation and survived, although his symptoms lasted for two days.[3] There are other reports of death in the medical literature due to ingestion of aconite-containing herbal remedies. Although accidental aconite poisoning is rare in North America, Pullela et al. presented a case in which a twenty-five-year-old man died suddenly following a recreational outing with his friends during which he ingested a number of wild berries and plants. One of the plants was later identified as monkshood. A high level of aconitine was found in his postmortem blood, confirming the cause of death as monkshood poisoning.[4]

Chan Su and Related Asian Medicines

The Chinese medicine Chan Su is prepared from the dried white secretion of the auricular and skin glands of Chinese toads (*Bufo melanostictus* or *Bufo bufo gargarizans*). Chan Su is also a major component of the traditional Chinese medicines Liu Shen Wan and Kyushin.[5] These medicines are used in China for the treatment of tonsillitis, sore throat, boils, palpitations, and other issues because of their anesthetic and antibiotic action. Traditional use of Chan Su given in small doses also includes stimulation of myocardial contraction, anti-inflammatory effects, and pain relief. The pharmacological effect of Chan Su is due to the actions of bufalin and cinobufagin, but bufalin is also very toxic. The death of a Chinese woman after ingestion of a Chinese herbal tea containing Chan Su has been reported.[6] Fortunately, Chan Su is not found in regular herbal stores and is sold only in selected Chinese herbal stores. Bufalin is structurally similar to digoxin, and an antidote of digoxin may be helpful in treating Chan-Su poisoning.[7]

> A twenty-three-year-old man died from heart failure after ingestion of a West Indian aphrodisiac known as "Love Stone." Chemical analysis showed the presence of the controlled substance bufotenine as well as bufalin and related compounds found in Chan Su.[8]

CASE STUDY

These cardioactive steroids from toad venom are dangerous and should be avoided under any circumstances.

Ephedra (Ma Huang)

Ephedra is a small perennial shrub with thin stems. Some of the better-known species include *Ephedra sinica* and *Ephedra equisetina* (collectively called Ma Huang). Ephedra contains many active compounds, such as pseudoephedrine, norephedrine, and phenylpropanolamine, with the predominant active compound being ephedrine, a potent stimulant of the central nervous system. Ephedrine can provide relief from cold and flu symptoms such as nasal congestion; it also constitutes approximately 1 percent of Ma Huang, a Chinese weight-loss product that contains ephedrine. Ma Huang is often referred to as the herbal alternative to fen-phen, the banned weight-loss drug containing fenfluramine. Sometimes "herbal fen-phen" products contain St. John's wort and are sold as "herbal Prozac." Ephedra-containing products are also marketed as decongestants, bronchodilators, and stimulants. Other promoted purposes include bodybuilding and enhancement of athletic performance. "Herbal Ecstasy," which can induce a euphoric state, also contains ephedrine.

Many reports of toxicity from ephedra-containing products have been published. Haller and Benowitz evaluated 140 reports of ephedra-related toxicity that were submitted to the FDA between June 1997 and 31 March 1999. They concluded that 31 percent of the cases were definitely related to ephedra toxicity and another 31 percent were possibly related. Of the reports of ephedra toxicity, 47 percent involved cardiovascular problems and 18 percent involved problems with the central nervous system. Hypertension was the single most frequent adverse reaction, followed by palpitation, tachycardia, stroke, and seizure. Ten events resulted in death and thirteen events caused permanent disability. The authors concluded that use of a dietary supplement that contains ephedra may pose a serious health risk.[9] Other than death, ephedra can increase blood pressure and cause cardiac arrhythmia and stroke. On 12 April 2004 the FDA prohibited the sale of ephedra-containing weight-loss supplements in the United States.[10] Exposure to ephedra alkaloid may also cause liver damage. Although banned in the United States, Ma Huang is available in Asian countries and is also used for treating colds, the flu, nasal congestion, asthma, and fever. The use of ephedra-containing products is also banned by the International Olympic Committee.

Hepatotoxic Herbs

Severe liver toxicity may result from the use of herbs such as chaparral, comfrey, germander, kava, mistletoe, and pennyroyal, as well as from the use of certain Chinese weight-loss products contaminated with aristolochic acid. (Please see Chapter 7 for a detailed discussion of these supplements.) Chinese medicines such as Jin Bu Huan, Ma Huang, and Sho Saiko are also known to cause severe liver toxicity and should be avoided. The hepatotoxicity of chaparral, germander, and other herbs (*Atractylis gummifera* and *Callilepsis laureola*) is due to the presence of pyrrolizidine alkaloids.[11] Several deaths have been reported due to use of the herbal sedative kava, and the FDA has warned consumers regarding use of this supplement. Severe liver toxicity requiring liver transplant in a sixty-year-old woman was related to taking chaparral for one year.[12] Gow et al. reported a case of fatality due to acute liver failure in a patient who ingested an herbal preparation containing kava and passionflower.[13]

> **CASE STUDY**
>
> A twenty-three-year-old man was admitted to the hospital due to liver failure (hepatic veno-occlusive disease). He ate a predominately vegetarian diet and was consuming comfrey leaves. The patient subsequently died from liver failure.[14]

Although comfrey was widely used in herbal supplements in the past, at present, oral herbal supplements containing comfrey are banned in the United States and the European Union. Comfrey is only available for topical application.

Pennyroyal oil is very toxic and should not be used. Sometimes it is used to induce abortion. It is very toxic to the liver, and its ingestion may cause death.[15] Fatal hepatitis in a sixty-eight-year-old woman was related to use of the herbal weight-loss product Tealine, which contained hepatotoxic germander extract.[16] Coltsfoot, another dangerous herbal supplement containing pyrrolizidine alkaloid, is often found in combination with other products and is used as a cough remedy. There are several reports of death in the medical literature due to the use of coltsfoot supplement.

> **CASE STUDY**
>
> Three women were admitted to the hospital with severe liver toxicity. They had been using an herbal tea and developed symptoms nineteen to forty-five days after they began use. Two patients stopped taking the tea, but the third patient continued, against medical advice, and eventually died. It was determined that the tea contained coltsfoot.

Death in an infant has also been reported following her mother drinking an herbal tea that contained coltsfoot.[17]

Methyl Salicylate/Oil of Wintergreen

Methyl salicylate is a major component of oil of wintergreen and is prepared by distillation from wintergreen leaves. Because of its analgesic effect it is used in many over-the-counter analgesic creams or gels for topical use. If ingested, it is very poisonous. Aspirin is acetyl salicylate, which is structurally close to methyl salicylate, but acetyl salicylate after ingestion rapidly breaks down into salicylic acid (the pain-relieving component of the chemical) in our blood and in the liver. In contrast, methyl salicylate is not broken down in our body to salicylic acid, which results in toxicity. Oil of wintergreen contains 98 percent methyl salicylate, and ingestion of 5 mL of oil of wintergreen (1 tsp) is equivalent to ingestion of 7,000 mg of aspirin. Methyl salicylate is a relatively common cause of child poisoning,[18] and for children under six years of age, oil of wintergreen in amounts of 1 tsp or less has been implicated in several well-documented deaths. The popular topical ointment Bengay contains 15 percent methyl salicylate, while Ultra Strength Bengay contains 30 percent. Many Chinese medicines and medicated oils, such as white flower oil and red flower oil, contain high amounts of methyl salicylate, and severe salicylate toxicity due to ingestion of these oils has been reported in adults, including one death due to ingestion of red-flower oil.[19]

CASE STUDY

Parker et al. reported another case, this time of a fifty-eight-year-old Vietnamese woman who lived alone in San Diego. Her brother discovered the body and called the emergency medical service. The paramedics confirmed death at the site, and police discovered a coffee cup containing a clear liquid with menthol odor and several empty medicine bottles, including one for a Chinese herbal medicine, on a bedside table. All of them were submitted to the medical examiner's office for investigation. High amounts of salicylic acid were found in the woman's blood and gastric content. The medicine bottles were identified as Koong Hung Yick Far oil, containing 67 percent oil of wintergreen, and Po Sum oil, containing 15 percent menthol. Methyl salicylate was also present in the gastric content, confirming that the cause of death was ingestion of methyl-salicylate–containing Chinese medicated oil.[20]

Poisoning from methyl salicylate can also occur due to abuse of topical cream containing methyl salicylate. Morra et al. demonstrated that after topical application of analgesic cream containing methyl salicylate, salicylic acid can be detected in the blood and the absorption rate of methyl salicylate increases after the first twenty-four hours of application and then steadily increases from the first to the seventh day.[21] In June 2007 the media reported that a seventeen-year-old athlete accidentally overdosed on an over-the-counter sports cream designed for treating sore muscles and joints. Although death from excessive use of a topical cream containing methyl salicylate is very rare, this case reminds us that these analgesic creams that provide relief from pain to millions of Americans may also have significant risk associated with overuse. Methyl salicylate is also fat-soluble, making it more toxic than aspirin. Common over-the-counter analgesic creams containing methyl salicylate are listed below.[22] Salicylate increases respiration and is followed by a severe imbalance of acid and base in the body (metabolic acidosis) that may cause death.

Brand Names of Some Common Over-the-Counter Analgesic Creams Containing Methyl Salicylate[23]

- ArthriCare
- Goanna Salve
- Icy Hot
- Massengill
- Pain Bust-R II
- Ultra Strength Bengay Cream
- Arthritis Formula Bengay Cream
- Gordogesic
- Listerine
- Minti-Rub
- Thera-Gesic

Oleander

The oleanders are flowering evergreen ornamental shrubs that belong to the dogbane family. They grow in southern parts of the United States (from Florida to California), Australia, India, Sri Lanka, China, and elsewhere. All parts of the oleander plant are toxic. Human exposure to oleander includes accidental ingestion, administration in food or drink, medicinal use (as herbal supplements), and criminal poisoning.[24] Despite its toxicity, oleander is still used in some folk medicines.[25] Boiling or drying the plant does not inactivate the toxins. A woman died after drinking herbal tea prepared from oleander.[26] Oleander contains oleandrin, which is similar in structure to the cardioactive drug digoxin and causes cardiac toxicity. Because of the structural similarity with digoxin, severe oleander poisoning can be treated with the same antidote (Digibind) used to treat digoxin poisoning. However, Digibind is expensive and there is a severe shortage of such antidotes in countries such as Sri Lanka.[27] If you live in southern sections of the United States, you are probably familiar with oleander trees and their beautiful flowers, but if you have small children, you should not even put this flower in your house, as oleander is frequently responsible for the accidental poisoning of children.

Thunder-God Vine

Thunder-god vine (Lei Gong Teng, prepared from the plant *Tripterygium wilfordii*) has been used in traditional Chinese medicine for more than two thousand years for local treatment of arthritis and inflamed tissue. It has also been indicated for treating rheumatoid arthritis. Unfortunately, thunder-god vine can cause severe adverse reactions and is poisonous if not carefully extracted from the skinned roots. Other parts of the plant, such as the leaves, flowers, and skin of the root, are very toxic to humans and may cause death if ingested.

CASE STUDY A thirty-six-year-old man was admitted to the hospital with severe diarrhea and vomiting that had lasted for three days. Three days before his admission, he had consumed an herbal supplement. He died fifteen hours after admission due to shock, hypotension (very low blood pressure), and cardiac damage. The herbal supplement the patient was taking was identified as thunder-god vine.[28]

Other Herbal and Natural Supplements You Should Avoid as Possibly Toxic

There are a few other herbs you should avoid because they are possibly toxic. A few of the more popular herbs in this category—bitter orange, guarana, and yohimbe—are widely used, so be sure to check the ingredients in your supplements carefully to make sure they aren't included.

Androstenedione

Androstenedione, a steroid produced by the body, is a common precursor of the male sex hormone testosterone and the female sex hormones estrogen, estradiol, and estrone. Androstenedione was manufactured and sold as a dietary supplement called "Andro" for improving performance in sports and for bodybuilding and weight loss. The FDA banned the sale of this dietary supplement in 2004, citing health risks, and sent letters to twenty-three companies asking them to stop distributing products sold as dietary supplements that contain androstenedione and warning them that they could face enforcement action if they did not.[29] Androstenedione can cause adverse cardiovascular reactions.[30]

Bitter Orange

Bitter orange, or Seville orange, has been used in traditional Chinese medicine, and today it is used mainly as a weight-loss product and as a nasal decongestant. It is also taken orally for the treatment of indigestion and nausea, and is applied topically to treat ringworm and athlete's foot. Following withdrawal of ephedrine from the marketplace of dietary supplements, weight-loss products containing bitter orange have been gaining popularity.

At this point, there is little evidence that bitter orange promotes weight loss. However, it contains synephrine and other compounds that are structurally similar to ephedrine. Ingestion of these herbal supplements may increase blood pressure and heart rate. Health Canada reported that from 1 January 1998 to 28 February 2004 it received sixteen reports in which products containing bitter orange or synephrine were suspected of being associated with adverse cardiovascular effects such as blackout, transient collapse, cardiac arrest, tachycardia, and ventricular fibrillation.[31] Bitter orange may cause resistant hypertension (high blood pressure). A fifty-five-year-old man who took 300 mg of bitter-orange extract every day had a heart attack (acute myocardial infarction). People with heart disease or high blood pressure should not take products containing bitter orange.[32] It should also be noted that bitter-orange oil, when applied to the skin, may cause photosensitive reactions.

Guarana

Guarana, a popular herbal weight-loss product—both by itself and as an ingredient in many herbal weight-loss compounds—is prepared from seeds of guarana containing 2.5–7 percent caffeine (200 mg/dose). In contrast, one cup of coffee contains 100 mg or less of caffeine. At the recommended dosage for weight loss, a person may take up to 1,800 mg of caffeine per day. Such high caffeine intake may produce adverse effects such as increasing blood pressure to a dangerous level in a person already suffering from high blood pressure. If a person taking such supplements also drinks coffee or takes any medicine such as pseudoephedrine, which may also increase blood pressure, there may be an additive effect on blood pressure, causing cardiac problems. A twenty-five-year-old woman with preexisting mitral-valve prolapse died from using an herbal supplement containing guarana and ginseng due to the high caffeine content of the herbal preparation.[33]

Lobelia

Lobelia (*Lobelia inflata*), also called Indian tobacco, has been used traditionally for the treatment of asthma and bronchitis. The leaves and seeds of lobelia are used in herbal remedies, and crude extract of lobelia has antidepressant activity, based on research using mice.[34] Unfortunately, lobelia is a potentially toxic herb, and ingestion may cause nausea, vomiting, rapid heartbeat, low blood pressure, and possibly coma. Therefore, it is advisable to avoid herbal supplements containing lobelia.

Nutmeg

Seeds of nutmeg are used as a spice, and nutmeg oil has many benefits, including an antibacterial effect. Historically, it was used as a stimulant and abortifacient, as well as to promote menstruation. Nutmeg also contains a volatile oil comprised of several active compounds, including myristicin, which is metabolized to an active compound with LSD-like effects. Due to its euphoric and hallucinogenic effects, nutmeg has long been used in large quantities as a low-cost substitute for other so-called recreational drugs. To obtain this effect, one must consume 15–20 g, which can produce severe toxicity. From 1998 to 2004, seventeen calls were made to the Texas Poison Center Network involving nutmeg poisoning, and eleven of the calls (all from males) were due to intentional abuse.[35] Stein et al. described a case in which a fifty-five-year-old woman died from nutmeg abuse, as confirmed by the presence of myristicin in the postmortem blood.[36] Toxicity may occur with ingestion of approximately 5 g of nutmeg, corresponding to 1 to 2 mg of myristicin, but it is very unlikely that intake of nutmeg as a spice would cause any toxicity because the amount of ingested myristicin and other active compounds would be very low.[37]

Pokeweed

Pokeweed (also known as American nightshade and *Phytolacca americana*) is a large perennial herb that can reach a height of ten to twelve feet and is found in California, Hawaii, Canada, and the eastern parts of North America, as well as in other parts of the world. The berries and dried roots are used for preparing herbal remedies and traditionally have been used by Native Americans to treat a variety of conditions, including skin disease, syphilis, cancer, and infections, and as an emetic and narcotic. Unfortunately, all parts of pokeweed are toxic. In the nineteenth century, poisonings from pokeweed were common in the United

States because pokeweed-root tinctures were used to treat rheumatism.[38] Eating uncooked berries also causes pokeweed poisoning. Although some people eat young leaves and berries (after cooking twice and discarding the water), there is no guarantee that such cooking makes pokeweed safe for human consumption. The toxicity of pokeweed increases with its maturity, but green berries are more toxic than red berries. There are several cases of pokeweed poisoning reported in the literature. It is advisable to avoid pokeweed-root tea and herbal supplements containing pokeweed.

Skullcap

Skullcap (*Scutellaria lateriflora*) is a native North American plant that has been used for centuries as a folk remedy to treat anxiety, nervous tension, and convulsions. It was once considered a remedy for rabies, but there is no scientific basis for this claim. It is mainly the leaves that are used in herbal remedies. Chinese skullcap (*Scutellaria baicalensis*) has anti-inflammatory, antiallergic, and many other pharmacological properties. Despite benefits, this herbal remedy probably should not be used due to several reports of toxicity, mainly to the liver. In one report, four women between ages forty-one and fifty-seven experienced severe jaundice after taking a skullcap-containing herbal remedy to relieve stress. Upon discontinuation of the supplement, their liver-function tests returned to normal in two to nineteen months.[39] There are other reports in the medical literature of liver toxicity due to the use of skullcap.

Wormwood

Herbal supplements containing wormwood or wormwood oil should be avoided because of the risk of neurological problems such as numbness of the leg, delirium, and even paralysis. Weisbord et al. reported seizure and acute renal failure in a thirty-one-year-old man who obtained wormwood essential oil through the Internet and drank 10 mL.[40]

Yohimbe

The bark of the yohimbe tree has traditionally been used in Africa to increase sexual desire and now is used as a dietary supplement for treating sexual dysfunction, including erectile dysfunction. Yohimbe bark can be brewed in tea or consumed as an extract that is available commercially. Although this supplement is effective in treating erectile dysfunction, its benefits seem to be outweighed by the risks.[41]

Yohimbe use has been associated with high blood pressure, increased heart rate, dizziness, and other symptoms, and if taken in large doses for a long time, it can be dangerous. A forty-three-year-old man died in a hotel room during sexual relations with a colleague. He was taking Viagra, and there were containers of several drugs in the room, including yohimbe.[42]

Conclusion

There are several herbal supplements available in health-food stores that may not be safe to consume. Although toxicities of most of these supplements are based on only a few case studies, in my opinion it would be wise to avoid them. Two case reports cited in *Consumer Reports* in May 2004 are good examples of how a dietary supplement perceived to be safe can cause serious adverse reactions. The article listed some toxic and potentially toxic herbal and natural supplements, including androstenedione, bitter orange, chaparral, comfrey, germander, kava, lobelia, pennyroyal oil, skullcap, and yohimbe, as well as Chinese dietary supplements containing aristolochic acid.[43] In a more recent *Consumer Reports* article, certain ingredients of dietary supplements, including cesium (a metal), colloidal silver, and organ/glandular extract were also listed as unsafe. The intended use of cesium is in controlling cancer and depression, while colloidal silver is intended to treat infection. Organ/glandular extract is indicated for fatigue or depression.[44]

In this chapter, all of the known toxic herbs have been discussed, but it is possible that in the future some herbs that are currently considered safe may indicate some specific toxicity. It is always best to discuss your choice of herbs with your physician, health-care provider, or a naturopathic doctor experienced with herbal supplements so that you can get benefits from an herb and avoid toxicity.

CHAPTER 9

How Herbal Remedies Interact with Your Medicines

Herbal remedies, like Western medicines, contain active ingredients, including complex chemical compounds produced by the plant through a process called biosynthesis. These active ingredients can have both beneficial and toxic effects. Health-care providers know that two Western drugs may interact with each other, causing drug toxicity or treatment failure. Similarly, an active component of an herbal remedy may interact with a Western medicine, causing harmful effects. In my first class in pharmacology, our professor told us, "Another name for medicine is poison. Please treat medicines with respect." For example, acetaminophen (Tylenol) is a common medication we take for pain control. Although we usually only take one or two tablets for a headache, if we were to take 10–15 tablets at once, it could cause severe liver damage and maybe even death. Medicines are not cakes, and we don't eat them as dessert. Herbal remedies, too, must be treated with respect. In this chapter, interactions of commonly used herbs with Western medications are discussed.

Drug-Drug and Drug-Herb Interaction

When one drug influences the effect of another drug, it is called drug-drug interaction. Similarly, when an herbal remedy influences the efficacy of a drug, it is called drug-herb interaction. Foods may have an effect on or interact with certain drugs, and alcohol should not be consumed when taking certain medications, since alcohol causes more of these drugs to be absorbed from the gut, with adverse effects. Conversely, certain foods induce the metabolism (i.e., speed up the conversion of a drug to a different form that enhances its excretion from the body) of certain drugs. This causes the drugs to move through the body and be excreted faster, and makes them less effective. It has been documented that smoking cigarettes and eating charcoal-broiled food and cruciferous vegetables (e.g., brussels sprouts, broccoli, cabbage, cauliflower, and radishes) induce the metabolism of several drugs, thus reducing their efficacy.

Drug-drug interactions can be broadly classified under two categories:

1. Pharmacokinetic interaction: This occurs when one drug affects the blood level and/or distribution of another drug by altering its absorption, metabolism, or excretion. The increased or decreased level of the affected drug in the blood alters its pharmacological effects, either reducing the therapeutic benefit or creating drug toxicity. For example, if a patient is taking digoxin for the treatment of heart disease and the physician prescribes an additional heart medicine such as quinidine, the dosage of digoxin must be reduced at least by half. Otherwise, the patient may experience toxicity because the concentration of digoxin in blood is increased by quinidine through a complex mechanism. As another example, drug A may displace drug B, preventing it from binding with its target protein receptors. This results in an increase in the unbound (free) fraction of drug B, which may cause toxicity. When valproic acid ("drug A"), a drug used in treating seizures, is given to a patient who is already taking the antiseizure medication phenytoin ("drug B"), the dosage of phenytoin must be adjusted because valproic acid displaces phenytoin from protein binding, thus increasing the free fraction of phenytoin.

2. Pharmacodynamic interaction: This occurs when one drug increases or decreases the action of another drug without altering its concentration in the blood. In general, two drugs with similar pharmacological actions, when used together, may have an additive effect, in which the combined effect is equal to the sum of the two drug's effects, or a synergistic effect, in which the combined effect is more than the sum of the pharmacological actions of each drug. One drug may also act as an antagonist to another drug, canceling its action.

Drug-herb interactions may be either pharmacokinetic or pharmacodynamic. St. John's wort, an herbal antidepressant, interacts pharmacokinetically with many medications by increasing their metabolism. Therefore, these drugs demonstrate less therapeutic benefits in patients also taking St. John's wort, due to reduced levels in the blood. St. John's wort also shows pharmacodynamic interaction with certain antidepressants such as SSRIs (selective serotonin reuptake inhibitors), producing excess serotonin in the central nervous system (CNS), which can cause serious drug toxicity (serotonin syndrome).

Many drug-herb interactions have been reported in various highly respected medical journals. Some are based on a single case report in which a patient experienced adverse effects due to drug interaction with herbal supplements, while others involve more rigorous studies, in which volunteers took certain drugs and herbs under controlled conditions.

Who Is Most Vulnerable to Drug-Herb Interactions?

Although drug-herb interactions can cause adverse effects in any patient, certain drug interactions with herbal products may result in medical emergency or even death.

CASE STUDY

In one study, Kupiec and Raj reported the case of a fifty-five-year-old man who was taking phenytoin and valproic acid to control seizures. The patient started taking herbal supplements, including ginkgo biloba (used to sharpen memory). The ginkgo interacted with both the phenytoin and the valproic acid, reducing their effectiveness by substantially decreasing their concentrations in the blood. In addition, the authors postulated that the ginkgo nut contains a potential neurotoxin that is known to induce seizures. The patient suffered a fatal breakthrough seizure; the authors speculate that he died due to the interaction of ginkgo with his medications.[1]

Certain groups of patients are at increased risk for drug toxicity due to potential drug-herb interaction and should avoid all herbal supplements unless approved by their doctors (see Table 9.1 on the next page). In addition, if you are taking any medication for the treatment of a chronic condition, please consult your doctor before using any herbal supplement.

TABLE 9.1: Patients Who Are Vulnerable to Drug-Herb Interaction

PATIENT GROUP	COMMENTS
AIDS patients	AIDS patients take multiple drugs, and interactions between their drugs and herbal supplements can result in treatment failure.
Patients with depression	Many medications used in treating depression interact with herbal remedies such as St. John's wort, kava, and valerian.
Diabetics	Several herbs decrease blood-sugar levels.
The elderly	Elderly patients may take multiple drugs for various chronic illnesses, making them especially susceptible to drug-herb interactions.
Heart patients	Various drugs used in treating cardiac dysfunction are very susceptible to interactions with herbs. In addition, many patients with heart problems may also take anticoagulants, which are very prone to drug-herb interaction.
Transplant recipients	To avoid rejection of the transplanted organ by the body, these patients need to take immunosuppressant drugs, which are prone to interactions with herbs, especially St. John's wort; a life-threatening situation may arise due to organ rejection.

Pregnant/nursing women should avoid all herbal supplements because some components of herbal supplements may cross the placenta or be secreted in milk and have adverse effects on the fetus.

What Are the Chances of Experiencing Drug-Herb Interactions?

Fortunately, only a fraction of over-the-counter and prescription medications account for most interactions with herbal supplements. In one study, Sood et al. surveyed 1,818 patients and identified 107 drug-herb interactions that had clinical significance. The five most common herbal supplements (St. John's wort, ginkgo, garlic, valerian, and kava) accounted for 68 percent of such interactions, and four classes of prescription drugs (antidepressants, antidiabetics, sedatives, and anticoagulants) accounted for 94 percent of all clinically significant interactions.[2] St. John's wort is responsible for many interactions with Western drugs.

One report identified thirty-two drugs that interact with herbal supplements.[3] Table 9.2 provides a list of drugs that are known to interact with various herbal supplements, broken down by the class of medication. If you are taking one of these drugs, it is wise not to take any herbal supplement without the approval of your physician.

TABLE 9.2: Drugs Known to Interact with Herbal Supplements

CLASS OF MEDICATION	DRUG
Analgesics	Acetaminophen, aspirin, ibuprofen, indomethacin, naproxen, tolmetin
Antiasthmatics	Theophylline
Anticancer drugs	Imatinib, irinotecan
Anticoagulants	Phenprocoumon, warfarin
Anticonvulsants	Phenobarbital, phenytoin
Antidepressants	Alprazolam, amitriptyline, fluoxetine, haloperidol, imipramine, midazolam, lithium, mirtazapine, nefazodone, paroxetine, phenelzine, sertraline, venlafaxine
Antidiabetics	Gliclazide, metformin, tolbutamide
Antihistamines	Fexofenadine
Anti-infectives	Erythromycin, voriconazole
Anti-Parkinson's drugs	Levodopa
Antiretrovirals	Atazanavir, indinavir, lamivudine, nevirapine, ritonavir, saquinavir
Cardioactive drugs	Digoxin, nifedipine, propanolol, verapamil
Cholesterol-lowering drugs	Atorvastatin, pravastatin, simvastatin
Cough suppressants	Dextromethorphan
Diuretics	Hydrochlorothiazide
Immunosuppressants	Cyclosporine, tacrolimus
Oral contraceptives	Ethinyl estradiol/desogestrel
Synthetic opioids (used in drug rehabilitation)	Methadone

The following is a list of common herbal products that interact with drugs. You may find it a broad list, but my firm position is that when it comes to drug-drug and drug-herb interactions, it is better to be safe than sorry. If you are taking any medication for the treatment of a chronic disease, please do not take any of these herbal products without first consulting with your health-care provider.

Nutritional Supplements Known to Interact with Drugs

- astragalus
- borage
- coenzyme Q10
- Dong Quai
- evening-primrose oil
- fish oil
- ginger
- black cohosh
- bromelain
- danshen
- echinacea
- feverfew
- garlic
- ginkgo biloba

- ginseng
- goldenseal
- hawthorn
- kelp
- milk thistle
- valerian
- glucosamine
- green tea
- kava
- licorice
- St. John's wort

How St. John's Wort Can Interact with Drugs

Research indicates that St. John's wort is as effective as tricyclic medications in treating patients with depression. The most commonly sold St. John's wort preparation in the United States is an alcoholic extract of hypericum, a perennial aromatic shrub with bright, yellow flowers that bloom from June to September. As mentioned previously, the flowers are most abundant and brightest around June 24th, the day traditionally believed to be the birthday of St. John the Baptist, hence the name St. John's wort. St. John's wort exhibits both pharmacokinetic and pharmacodynamic interactions with various drugs.

If you are taking any medication for any chronic condition, please do not take St. John's wort.

Pharmacokinetic Interactions

Many Western drugs are metabolized by a family of specialized enzymes in the liver known collectively as cytochrome P-450 (CYP-450)* mixed-function oxidase. Enzymes are basically proteins, and CYP-450 enzymes are called hemoproteins because they contain iron molecules. (Hemoglobin, which is responsible for carrying oxygen in the blood and which produces the blood's red color, is also a hemoprotein.) CYP-450 enzymes are found in many forms of life, including birds, fish, worms, plants, fungus, and mammals. More than two hundred drugs and many endogenous compounds (compounds found in or produced by the body) such as estrogen, progesterone, and testosterone are metabolized by CYP-450. Many drugs, carbamazepine, for example, induce CYP-450 and thus increase the metabolism of drugs that are metabolized by these enzymes. Therefore, the drug becomes less effective due to increased metabolism, and it is excreted faster from

* The name cytochrome P-450 is derived from the fact that these enzymes are colored (Greek word *chrome*), cellular (*cyto*) proteins that show an absorption peak in spectrum at 450 nm wavelength when the iron in the molecule is reduced (loses an electron).

the body, reducing its concentration in the blood. Because the pharmacological activity of a drug depends on its blood concentration, a lower drug concentration in the blood reduces the drug's efficacy.

The active components of St. John's wort, and especially hyperforin, induce CYP-450 enzymes by a complex mechanism. Hypericin, another component of St. John's wort, induces other complex molecules known as drug transporters, which may affect the concentration of certain drugs in the blood, causing treatment failure. Published reports in medical journals indicate that St. John's wort significantly reduces blood concentrations of many drugs due to increased metabolism of the drugs by the liver.[4] Therefore self-medication with St. John's wort may cause treatment failure due to a reduced concentration of a drug in the blood. Important pharmacokinetic interactions of drugs with St. John's wort are listed in Table 9.3.

TABLE 9.3: Drugs That Have Pharmacokinetic Interactions with St. John's Wort

CLASS OF MEDICATION	DRUG
Antiasthmatics	Theophylline
Anticancer drugs	Imatinib, irinotecan
Anticoagulants (blood thinners)	Warfarin
Anticonvulsants	Phenobarbital, phenytoin
Antidepressants	Amitriptyline
Antidiabetic drugs	Gliclazide, tolbutamide
Anti-inflammatories	Fexofenadine, ibuprofen
Antimicrobials (used in treating bacterial or fungal infections)	Erythromycin (bacterial), voriconazole (fungal)
Anti-Parkinson's drugs	Levodopa
Antiretrovirals (Used in treating patients with AIDS)	Atazanavir, indinavir, lamivudine, nevirapine, saquinavir
Benzodiazepines (sedatives/anti-anxiety drugs)	Alprazolam, midazolam
Cardioactive drugs	Digoxin, nifedipine, verapamil
Cough suppressants	Dextromethorphan
Immunosuppressants (used in transplant recipient to avoid organ rejection)	Cyclosporine, tacrolimus
Oral contraceptives	Estrogen, progestin
Proton-pump inhibitors (for acid reflux)	Omeprazole
Statins (cholesterol-lowering drugs)	Atorvastatin, pravastatin
Synthetic opioids	Methadone

The drugs listed in Table 9.4 have no known interaction with St. John's wort.

TABLE 9.4: Drugs with No Known Interactions with St. John's Wort

CLASS OF MEDICATION	DRUG
Antiepileptics	Carbamazepine
Immunosuppressants	Mycophenolic acid

A transplant recipient may face acute organ rejection due to self-medication with St. John's wort because St. John's wort reduces the efficacy of immunosuppressant drugs such as cyclosporine and tacrolimus, which the transplant recipient takes for life to prevent organ rejection. St. John's wort results in faster metabolism of both drugs by the liver and can reduce their blood concentrations by more than 50 percent. Based on actual case studies involving transplant recipients, it was concluded that St. John's wort can endanger the success of an organ transplant.[5]

Warfarin (brand name Coumadin) is used for thinning blood so that blood-clot formation (thrombosis) or the migration of a blood clot (embolism) can be avoided. This drug is used to treat a variety of conditions, including heart disease. Warfarin therapy should be carefully controlled by measuring the clotting capacity of blood, since overaction (too much thinning) may cause death due to excessive bleeding and undercoagulation may produce a fatal blood clot. St. John's wort diminishes the anticoagulant effect of warfarin by increasing its metabolism by liver enzymes.[6] A patient attending a Coumadin clinic (clinics in which patients taking the blood thinner Coumadin are monitored to make sure a blood clot is not formed) must avoid St. John's wort because failure of warfarin therapy may have significant clinical implications.

Protease inhibitors are a relatively new class of antiretroviral drugs that are very effective in treating patients with AIDS. A combination (cocktail) of these drugs, along with other, older drugs, produces lifesaving result in AIDS patients. Unfortunately, St. John's wort greatly reduces the efficacy of protease inhibitors such as indinavir, lopinavir, saquinavir, and atazanavir by inducing their metabolism, causing treatment failure. In addition, other retroviral agents such as lamivudine and nevirapine are negatively affected by St. John's wort. Treatment failure can result in a mutation of HIV, and the mutated virus may no longer respond to the drug cocktail.

> *In order to avoid treatment failure, patients taking immunosuppressant drugs (cyclosporine, tacrolimus), warfarin, or antiretrovirals should not take St. John's wort or any herbal supplement without consulting their doctor or pharmacist.*

St. John's wort may inactivate the effect of oral contraceptives. It increases the activities of the liver enzymes that metabolize oral contraceptives, reducing the effective concentration of them in the blood.

Omeprazole, a proton-pump inhibitor used in treating acid reflux, prevents the stomach from secreting excess hydrochloric acid, which may cause heartburn and other symptoms. St. John's wort inactivates omeprazole by increasing its metabolism.

St. John's wort reduces the efficacy of simvastatin, a cholesterol-lowering drug, thus increasing risk for heart disease.

Although St. John's wort has antidepressant effects, it reduces the efficacy of the antidepressant amitriptyline by reducing blood levels of the drug. In addition, St. John's wort reduces the effectiveness of many other drugs including digoxin, fexofenadine, methadone, midazolam, phenprocoumon, phenytoin, verapamil, and theophylline.[7]

Herbal remedies are not prepared following rigorous standards, and concentrations of active ingredients may vary among different manufacturers or even among batches of the remedy produced by the same manufacturer. St. John's wort containing low concentrations of hyperforin (less than 1 percent) may not cause pharmacokinetic interactions with Western drugs. It takes about two weeks of continuous use of St. John's wort before clinically significant interactions with drugs are observed. After discontinuation of St. John's wort, it also takes about two weeks for blood levels of the drug to return to what they were previously.

Pharmacodynamic Interactions

Although pharmacokinetic interactions of drugs with St. John's wort are more common, there are also important pharmacodynamic interactions. St. John's wort exerts its antidepressant effect by inhibiting uptake of serotonin, norepinephrine, and dopamine (chemicals known as neurotransmitters). Hyperforin, an active component of St. John's wort, is responsible for this effect. Many antidepressant drugs work through the same basic mechanism. Therefore, if a patient takes an antidepressant such as fluoxetine, sertraline, or paroxetine (all SSRIs, selective serotonin reuptake inhibitors), or imipramine or venlafaxine (which inhibit uptake of both serotonin and norepinephrine), along with St. John's wort, serotonin levels in the neurons will be highly elevated, causing drug toxicity known as "serotonin syndrome." The clinical symptoms include severe restlessness, muscle twitching, sweating, shivering, penile erection, tremor, and even seizure and coma.[8]

Table 9.5 lists other drugs that may have pharmacodynamic interactions with St. John's wort.

TABLE 9.5: Pharmacodynamic Drug Interactions with St. John's Wort

CLASS OF MEDICATION	DRUG
Antidepressants	Lithium, mirtazapine, monoamine oxidase inhibitors, venlafaxine
Central nervous system stimulants	Diethylpropion, phentermine
Drugs of abuse	Amphetamines, cocaine, ecstasy (3,4-methylenedioxy-methamphetamine), LSD (lysergic acid diethylamide)

Possible Interactions of Warfarin and Herbal Supplements

Warfarin has clinically significant interactions with various herbal supplements. Pharmacokinetic interactions occur with St. John's wort (see above) and with milk thistle. Because milk thistle inhibits liver enzymes, this interaction increases the effectiveness of warfarin. There are also pharmacodynamic interactions between herbal supplements and warfarin. Warfarin is derived from a naturally occurring compound (coumarin) found in plants. Many herbal supplements contain coumarin and thus may exert additive effects with warfarin, causing excessive anticoagulation.

Although the concentration of warfarin is usually not measured in clinical therapy, warfarin therapy is closely monitored in clinical laboratories by measuring INR (international normalization ratio). Warfarin's anticoagulant effect increases (which may cause excessive bleeding) if it is combined with coumarin-containing herbal remedies such as fenugreek, boldo, and Dong Quai or with anti-platelet herbs such as danshen, garlic, and ginkgo biloba. The INR was increased (indicating increased effect of warfarin) in a patient treated with warfarin for atrial fibrillation when he started taking boldo and fenugreek. After discontinuation of the herbal supplements, his INR returned to normal after one week. Consumption of coenzyme Q10 and ginger also appears to increase the risk of bleeding during warfarin therapy. In addition, both green tea and green, leafy vegetables (e.g., turnip greens, broccoli, lettuce, cabbage, spinach, and green beans) inhibit the action of warfarin. These vegetables (especially turnip greens and broccoli) are rich in vitamin K, and warfarin acts by inhibiting the action of vitamin K that participates in the clotting of blood.[9]

Various nutritional supplements such as fish oil (which contains omega-3 fatty acids) and Evening-primrose oil (which contains gamma-linoleic acid) also have pharmacodynamic interaction with warfarin. Table 9.6 lists herbal and nutritional supplements that interact with warfarin.[10]

TABLE 9.6: Herbal Products and Nutritional Supplements That Interact with Warfarin Therapy

HERBAL PRODUCT/ NUTRITIONAL SUPPLEMENT	EFFECT ON WARFARIN
Boldo	Increased
Borage	Increased
Coenzyme Q10	Increased
Danshen	Increased
Devil's claw	Increased
Dong Quai	Increased
Evening-primrose oil	Increased
Fenugreek	Increased
Feverfew	Increased
Fish oil	Increased
Garlic	Increased
Ginkgo biloba	Increased
Goldenseal	Reduced
Grape seed	Increased
Green tea	Reduced
Horse chestnut	Increased
Milk thistle	Reduced
Papaya	Increased
Royal jelly	Increased
Saw palmetto	Increased
St. John's wort	Reduced
Vitamin E	Increased

Although you should not take garlic, ginger, or fenugreek supplements
if you are receiving warfarin therapy, use of fenugreek, garlic, or ginger
in food is fine. The supplements contain much higher amounts of active
ingredients than you get in food. Fish oil supplements should be avoided
if you are on warfarin therapy, but eating fish up to two to three times a
week is okay.

Possible Drug Interactions with Ginkgo Biloba

Ginkgo biloba is prepared from dried leaves of the ginkgo tree through organic extraction (acetone/water). After the solvent is removed, the extract is dried and standardized. Most commercial-dosage forms contain 40 mg of extract. Ginkgo biloba is sold in the United States as a dietary supplement for sharpening mental focus and to improve diabetes-related circulatory disorder. In Germany, ginkgo is approved for improving memory and for treating depression, dizziness, vertigo, and headache. Ginkgo leaf contains various complex organic compounds including several glycosides (ginkgolide A and B), which are potent antagonists of platelet activity factor and also have antioxidant effects. As mentioned earlier, ginkgo biloba should not be taken with the blood thinner warfarin because it increases the effect of warfarin and may cause excessive bleeding.

Ginkgo biloba induces cytochrome P-450 liver enzymes and increases the metabolism of many drugs, causing treatment failure. In one study using eighteen healthy subjects, the authors observed that serum concentrations of omeprazole and omeprazole sulfone (metabolite of omeprazole) were significantly reduced following treatment with ginkgo biloba. One case report indicated fatal seizures in a fifty-five-year-old male, possibly due to the interaction of ginkgo biloba with the antiepileptic drugs phenytoin and valproic acid. The patient suffered a fatal breakthrough seizure with no evidence of noncompliance with anticonvulsant medications (these drugs are routinely monitored in blood to ensure their effectiveness and also to avoid drug toxicity). The postmortem blood concentrations of both drugs were extremely low compared with the levels prior to his death. The authors postulated that this fatal drug-herb interaction occurred because of rapid metabolism of phenytoin and valproic acid due to induction of liver enzymes by ginkgo biloba. Another report indicated that two patients who were stable with valproic acid developed seizures within two weeks of using ginkgo products. After discontinuing the use of ginkgo, both patients were again seizure-free without any increases in dose of valproic acid.

Animal studies using rats indicate reduced blood concentrations of cyclosporine when ginkgo biloba is administered. Moreover, experiments using rats also demonstrate that ginkgo biloba extract reduces the hypotensive (blood pressure-lowering) effect of nicardipine and the hypoglycemic (blood sugar level–lowering) effect of tolbutamide.[11]

There are reports describing bleeding associated with the use of ginkgo biloba. Bent et al. found fifteen published case reports describing an association between using ginkgo biloba and a bleeding event. Most cases reported involved serious medical conditions; six reports clearly demonstrated that after discontinuation of ginkgo, bleeding did not recur.[12]

> *Patients with bleeding disorders should not take ginkgo biloba. Moreover, if you are taking aspirin or another nonsteroidal anti-inflammatory drug, please consult with your doctor before taking ginkgo biloba. Use of ginkgo biloba must be discontinued at least two weeks before elective surgery in order to avoid the risk of excessive bleeding.*

Possible Drug Interactions with Ginseng

There are different types of ginseng; Asian ginseng, Siberian ginseng, Korean ginseng, and American ginseng are the most widely used. The Chinese ginseng that grows in Manchuria is *Panax ginseng*. However, the ginseng that grows in North America is a different species (*Panax quinquefolius*).

Human studies demonstrate that Asian ginseng (*Panax ginseng*), the most popular ginseng used in the United States, can lower blood alcohol levels. The most common preparation of ginseng is ginseng root extract. All types of ginseng have a psychoactive effect and show pharmacodynamic interaction with phenelzine, a monoamine oxidase inhibitor, causing serious toxicity and mania (due to an additive effect).[13] *Panax ginseng* may interact with caffeine to cause hypertension. All types of ginseng may also decrease the efficacy of warfarin. The analgesic effect of opioid medications (codeine, oxycodone) may be lost if taken with ginseng. [14] Ginseng, and especially ginseng metabolites, may inhibit cytochrome P-450 liver enzymes, thus reducing clearance of certain drugs and increasing their blood levels. Ginseng may also lower blood sugar and should not be taken by anyone with diabetes or by anyone being treated with any hypoglycemic agents. In addition, aspirin and related NSAIDS (ibuprofen-containing drugs such as Advil and Motrin) should not be taken with ginseng. If you are taking any of the drugs listed in Table 9.7, you should avoid taking ginseng.

TABLE 9.7: Drugs That Interact with Ginseng

CLASS OF MEDICATION	DRUG
Anticoagulants	Heparin, warfarin
Hypoglycemics	Chloropyramine, glipizide, glyburide, insulin, metformin, rosiglitazone, tolbutamide
Nonsteroidal anti-inflammatories	Aspirin, ibuprofen, indomethacin, ketoprofen, naproxen, tolmetin
Psychoactives	Phenelzine

Possible Drug Interactions with Kava

Kava, an herbal remedy that has both sedative and calming effects, has possible damaging and toxic effects, which were discussed in Chapters 7 and 8. It is prepared from a South Pacific plant (*Piper methysticum*), and a kava drink is prepared by mixing fresh or dried root with cold water or coconut milk. The neurological effects of kava are probably related to a group of compounds called kava lactones. These inhibit cytochrome P-450 liver enzymes and thus the metabolism of certain drugs, potentially causing drug toxicity. The most important interactions of kava with drugs are pharmacodynamic in nature. It is speculated that kava interacts with central nervous system (CNS) depressants such as benzodiazepines, alcohol, and barbiturates.

CASE STUDY

A fifty-four-year-old patient taking alprazolam, cimetidine, and terazosin started self-medication with kava for three days and was hospitalized. The authors suggested that kava lactones and alprazolam used together have additive effects because both act on the same GABA (gamma-aminobutyric acid) receptors. Moreover, kava lactones inhibit the metabolism of alprazolam and increase its level in the blood, causing toxicity.[15]

Possible Drug Interactions with Valerian

Valerian is a popular herbal sedative that acts by dose-dependent release (the amount of neurotransmitter released depends on the dosage of valerian taken) of the neurotransmitter gamma-aminobutyric acid (GABA) in the brain. Because many sedatives and antipsychotic drugs act by similar mechanisms, valerian can have additive effects when used with these drugs, resulting in severe drug toxicity. Valerian increases the sedative effect of midazolam and other benzodiazepines and barbiturates. It also prolongs thiopental- and pentobarbital-induced sleep. A potentially adverse interaction between haloperidol and valerian has been reported.[16]

Other Miscellaneous Drug-Herb Interactions

Echinacea is a popular herbal supplement used for boosting the immune system and preventing colds and other upper-respiratory-tract infections. It should be avoided if taking immunosuppressant drugs such as cyclosporine. In addition, echinacea may be toxic to the liver, especially if used with acetaminophen, other hepatotoxic drugs, or the anticancer drug methotrexate.

Astragalus, another popular immunomodulatory herbal supplement, should be avoided when taking cyclosporine, azathioprine, and methotrexate.

Black cohosh, red clover, and Dong Quai are commonly used herbal remedies for the alleviation of symptoms of menopause. These remedies contain hormones of plant origin (phytoestrogens) and may interfere with hormone replacement therapy (HRT), which itself may be contraindicated based on the results of the famous WHI HRT study, which was stopped in July of 2002 because the results indicated that HRT might increase a woman's risk of breast cancer, heart disease, blood clots, and stroke. Black cohosh may also be toxic to the liver. Dong Quai increases the effect of warfarin and should not be taken if on warfarin therapy.

Black pepper can inhibit cytochrome P-450, thus inducing drug toxicity. Both black and red pepper increased blood concentrations of phenytoin, propanolol, and theophylline.[17]

Licorice is commonly taken to alleviate symptoms of ulcers. Because it tends to increase blood pressure, it should be avoided by anyone being treated for hypertension. Licorice may also increase loss of potassium from the body and may interfere with diuretics (hydrochlorothiazide and related drugs).

Goldenseal also interacts with antihypertensive medicines and should therefore be avoided by anyone taking medication to control high blood pressure.

Hawthorn is used to treat heart disease and should not be taken in combination with any cardioactive drug such as digoxin. Similarly, many Chinese herbs indicated for treating heart conditions interact with cardioactive drugs and should not be taken at the same time. Guggul reduces the efficacy of beta-blockers and calcium channel blockers used in treating various conditions, including heart disease.

Ginger root and goldenseal may increase stomach-acid secretion and should be avoided by anyone who suffers from acidity or acid reflux and by anyone who is taking acid-suppression medication such as omeprazole.

Ipriflavone is made from soy and is sold as a dietary supplement. This supplement may have bone-protecting effects. However, it can increase the effects of theophylline, warfarin, and diabetic medications, causing toxicity. People with liver or kidney problems should also avoid this supplement.

Kelp, as a source of iodine, may interfere with thyroid replacement therapies. Licorice may offset the pharmacological action of spironolactone.

NSAIDS such as aspirin have the potential to interact with herbal supplements that can inhibit the aggregation of platelets in the blood. They can also interact with coumarin-containing herbs (e.g., chamomile, fenugreek, horse chestnut), which can also prevent blood coagulation.

Many herbs such as ginseng and karela, as well as supplements such as chromium, may significantly lower blood glucose.[18]

Miscellaneous drug-herb interactions are listed in Table 9.8.

TABLE 9.8: Other Miscellaneous Drug-Herb Interactions

HERBAL/ NUTRITIONAL SUPPLEMENT	INTERACTING DRUGS	EFFECT
Bromelain	Naproxen	Increased bleeding
Coenzyme Q10	Hydrochlorothiazide, metformin, glipizide	Hypotension, hypoglycemia
Garlic	Chlorpropamide, ibuprofen, saquinavir	Bleeding, decrease in efficacy of a drug, hypoglycemia
Ginkgo biloba	Aspirin, clopidogrel, dipyridamole, phenytoin, ticlopidine, trazodone, valproic acid	Bleeding, coma, reduced effects

(cont'd.)

TABLE 9.8: Other Miscellaneous Drug-Herb Interactions (cont'd.)

HERBAL/ NUTRITIONAL SUPPLEMENT	INTERACTING DRUGS	EFFECT
Echinacea	Ketoconazole, lansoprazole, methotrexate, simvastatin	Liver toxicity, increased effects
Feverfew	Azathioprine, cyclosporine, iron, tacrolimus	Reduced absorption, reduced immunosuppression
Fish oil	Metoprolol	Hypotension
Flaxseed oil	Aspirin	Increased bleeding
Glucosamine	Acetaminophen, glyburide	Decrease in efficacy of a drug, hyperglycemia
Kava	Alprazolam, benzodiazepines	Coma
Licorice	Atenolol	Hypotension
Milk thistle	Warfarin	Increased bleeding
Saw palmetto	Aspirin	Bleeding
Valerian	Barbiturates, midazolam	Increased sedation

Conclusion

There are many drug-herb interactions, and such interactions are either pharmacokinetic or pharmacodynamic in nature. Pharmacokinetic drug-herb interactions occur when a particular herbal supplement induces or inhibits drug-metabolizing enzymes. St. John's wort is known for many reported drug-herb interactions because some of its components induce liver enzymes and thus increase the metabolism of many drugs, causing therapeutic failure. If you are taking any Western medicines (prescription or over-the-counter), please avoid St. John's wort or take it only with the approval of your physician.

> *Treat herbal supplements with respect, and if you are taking any medication for a chronic condition, please do not take any herbal product without your physician's approval.*

There are also many reported pharmacodynamic interactions between herbs and drugs. Acetaminophen may produce liver toxicity if taken with herbal supplements like kava and echinacea. Unfortunately, drug-herb interactions can be very dangerous.[19]

CHAPTER 10

Food, Alcohol, Fruit Juices, Smoking — and Your Meds

If you look at your medications, you will notice that some labels tell you to take the medication on an empty stomach, while others tell you to take it with food, or that alcohol should not be consumed while you are taking the particular drug. In this chapter, we will discuss the rationales behind these guidelines. For example, several fruit juices, particularly grapefruit juice, *increase* absorption of drugs from the stomach and may cause drug toxicity, so this chapter will inform you about which fruit juices to avoid if you are taking certain medications.

Food-Drug Interactions

It has long been recognized that the intake of food and fluid can alter our ability to absorb drugs. Food-drug interactions may either increase the absorption of a drug, thus potentially increasing its adverse effects, or decrease absorption, reducing its efficacy. These effects of increasing or decreasing the absorption of drugs may be related to an alteration of physiological factors in the gut such as gastric acidity, gastric emptying time, and intestinal motility (the intestines' ability to contract and move food and waste through them). In addition, the rate of blood flow in the liver, or bile-flow rate, may also affect how much of the drug goes into the bloodstream. Moreover, direct interaction of food with a drug may alter absorption of the drug. For example, if a drug becomes trapped in the insoluble component of dietary fat, then lesser amounts are absorbed. In addition, food may alter the performance of extended-release medications.[1]

The first reported food-drug interaction was that of cheese and certain drugs. It has also been demonstrated that smoking and the intake of charcoal-broiled food or cruciferous vegetables (e.g., broccoli, cauliflower, cabbage) can increase the metabolism of several drugs, thus decreasing their blood concentrations and efficacy. In a study using six volunteers, Fegan et al. observed increased removal of propranolol (a blood pressure–lowering drug) and theophylline (an antiasthmatic) from the body when a high-protein, low-carbohydrate diet was consumed, compared with a low-protein, high-carbohydrate diet. Therefore, a high-protein, low-carbohydrate diet reduces efficacy of both propanolol and theophylline.[2]

The individuals who are most vulnerable to food-drug interactions are the elderly, patients with cancer, AIDS patients, transplant recipients, and patients with absorption problems. Certain drugs *should* be taken after meals because food intake stimulates the gastric juices and may help to dissolve the drugs, thus facilitating their absorption. These drugs include amoxicillin and cefuroxime (antibiotics), the cholesterol-lowering drug lovastatin, and lithium (an antipsychotic).[3] Commonly used over-the-counter analgesics (NSAIDS) such as aspirin, ibuprofen, naproxen, and prescription medications including tolmetin, mefenamic acid, and indomethacin should be taken with food or milk to avoid gastric irritation. On the other hand, the antibiotic tetracycline should *not* be taken with milk, which reduces its effectiveness.

While food intake increases absorption of certain drugs, it decreases absorption in many others due to a number of factors. Drugs such as furosemide (a diuretic) may bind to food and become ineffective. The antimalarial drug chloroquine is not absorbed in the presence of milk because milk contains calcium, and calcium binds to the drug. Digoxin, used in treating heart conditions, may not be absorbed if a meal with high fiber content is eaten. A high-protein meal may reduce absorption of levodopa, which is used in treating patients suffering from Parkinson's disease.[4]

Monoamine oxidase inhibitors (MAOIs), used for treating various psychiatric illnesses, are affected by specific foods. Monoamine oxidase, an enzyme in the digestive tract, metabolizes tyramine, an amino acid that is found in foods at a safe level. The amount of tyramine necessary to increase blood pressure is small, and if the activity of monoamine oxidase is inhibited (its biological activity is partially impaired), the tyramine level in the blood can increase, because tyramine is not being metabolized properly by the inactivated monoamine oxidase. This excess tyramine can cause severe hypertension, which may even lead to coma and death. Tyramine is found in small amounts in many foods but in higher levels in aged cheese, aged meat, fish, soybean products, tap beers, and red wine.[5] Isoniazid, which is used in treating tuberculosis, is also a weak monoamine oxidase inhibitor and has known interactions with aged cheese, wine, and other foods high in tyramine.

Folic acid increases clearance of phenytoin, increasing the chance of seizure in patients taking this medication. Wheat, flour, and cereals are fortified with folic acid, and it is also found in black-eyed peas, pinto beans, raw spinach, orange juice, pineapple juice, etc. Black pepper decreases the metabolism of phenytoin. Foods containing vitamin K are known to reduce the effectiveness of warfarin and may cause blood clotting. High amounts of vitamin K are found in leafy vegetables such as spinach, cabbage, kale, cauliflower, broccoli, and brussels sprouts, and in fruits such as avocado and kiwi. Parsley also contains a significant amount of vitamin K.

Important food-drug interactions are summarized in Table 10.1. This list is representative, not complete. The drugs listed are widely prescribed and it is important to know their medical recommendations, most of which are found on the labels of the medications. Please read each of your medication labels carefully to determine whether you should take the drug on an empty stomach, two hours after a meal, or with food. Your doctor and pharmacist are also very good resources and can give you proper guidance on getting the maximum benefits from your medication.

TABLE 10.1: Important Food-Drug Interactions

Drug	Recommendations
Ampicillin, azithromycin, chloroquine, ciprofloxacin, digoxin, erythromycin, isoniazid, iron, itraconazole, levodopa, tacrolimus	Do not take within two hours of a meal
Aspirin, amoxicillin, cimetidine, cefuroxime, ibuprofen, indomethacin, lovastatin, lithium, naproxen, nifedipine, tolmetin, ranitidine, saquinavir, zidovudine	Do not take with food
Doxycycline, tetracycline	Do not take with milk or food
Isoniazid, monoamine oxidase inhibitors	Avoid food high in tyramine
Phenytoin	Avoid folic acid and black pepper
Suxamethonium	Avoid tomatoes/potatoes
Warfarin	Avoid charcoal-grilled meats, avocado, and other food high in vitamin K

High amounts of vitamin K are found in leafy vegetables and also in liver. If you are taking warfarin, do not abruptly change your diet and increase intake of these foods in more quantities without discussing it with your physician. Also, do not take aspirin and related over-the-counter analgesics (nonsteroidal anti-inflammatory drugs) without the approval of your physician in order to avoid any risk of bleeding.

Alcohol-Drug Interactions

Alcohol is known to interact with certain drugs and should be avoided if these medications are taken. Two types of alcohol-drug interactions are observed. In a pharmacokinetic interaction, alcohol interferes with the absorption or metabolism of medications. In a pharmacodynamic interaction, alcohol enhances the effect of medication, particularly medications that produce dizziness, drowsiness, and sedation.[6] Drinking alcohol (a single drink or several drinks over hours) may inhibit (impair) the metabolism of a drug, causing drug toxicity. On the other hand, in alcoholics, a drug may not act well due to a complex interaction between excessive alcohol and the damaged liver. Some medications such as cough syrup and laxatives may contain as much as 10 percent alcohol. Women are more susceptible to alcohol than men; in general, if a woman consumes the same amount of alcohol as a man she will have a higher alcohol blood level. Elderly people are also more prone to adverse effects from alcohol interacting with their drugs and medications compared to the general healthy population.

Probably the most important drug-alcohol interaction results in liver damage. Acetaminophen (Tylenol), a common over-the-counter drug, can damage the liver if taken with alcohol for several days. It is well documented in the medical literature that alcoholics are very susceptible to severe liver damage even if they take the recommended dosage of acetaminophen. In one study, the authors treated six chronic alcoholics who developed severe liver toxicity when they took acetaminophen in moderate doses. The authors also identified nineteen other cases from the medical literature and concluded that liver damage in these patients was due to acetaminophen-alcohol interactions.[7] Wootton and Lee reported from a retrospective review (a review of cases after treatments have been completed) of seven alcoholics who had severe acute liver damage soon after using acetaminophen for therapeutic purposes; three patients died.[8]

Individuals taking cholesterol-lowering medications such as various statins or niacin are also at increased risk for liver damage if they regularly consume alcohol. In general, these medications have a tendency to cause liver damage. If you are taking such medications, your physician should require a liver-function test every six months. Fluconazole, a drug used in treating fungal infections, and isoniazid, used to treat tuberculosis, may also cause liver damage if combined with alcohol. Table 10.2 lists identifies drugs that interact with alcohol and the resulting effects.

TABLE 10.2: Important Alcohol-Drug Interactions

CLASS OF MEDICATION	DRUG	INTERACTION
Allergy and cold medications, cough suppressants	Chlorpheniramine, desloratadine, dextromethorphan, diphenhydramine, fexofenadine, loratadine	Increased dizziness
Analgesics	Acetaminophen, ibuprofen, naproxen	Liver damage, stomach upset, ulcer, bleeding
Antiangina drugs	Isosorbide, nitroglycerin	Rapid heartbeat, dizziness, fainting
Antianxiety drugs/ antidepressants	Alprazolam (Xanax), amitriptyline, citalopram, clonazepam, desipramine, diazepam, fluoxetine (Prozac), lorazepam, paroxetine (Paxil), sertraline (Zoloft), trazodone, venlafaxine	Drowsiness, dizziness, risk of overdose
Antidiabetic drugs	Metformin (Glucophage), glyburide (Micronase), tolbutamide (Orinase)	Abnormally low blood sugar
Antihypertensives	Benazepril (Lotensin), clonidine, enalapril, hydrochlorothiazide, losartan, quinapril (Accupril), prazosin	Drowsiness, dizziness, fainting
Anti-infectives	Metronidazole (Flagyl), cycloserine, tinidazole, nitrofurantoin, ketoconazole, isoniazid	Fast heartbeat, sudden change in blood pressure, upset stomach, liver damage
Blood thinners	Warfarin	Internal bleeding with alcohol consumption; clot formation in chronic drinkers
Cholesterol-lowering drugs	Lovastatin, atorvastatin (Lipitor), pravastatin, simvastatin (Zocor), niacin	Liver damage
Severe pain relief drugs	Hydrocodone (Vicodin), oxycodone (Percocet), propoxyphene	Increased risk of overdose
Sleeping aids	Zolpidem (Ambien), estazolam, temazepam, diphenhydramine, doxylamine	Drowsiness, impaired motor control

When combined with certain drugs, even small amounts of alcohol may impair motor skills, making it difficult to drive. Consumption of alcohol with some medications such as antianxietals, antidepressants, and even over-the-counter cold and flu medications may make you dizzy and drowsy. Operating heavy machinery or driving may be dangerous under such circumstances.

The interaction between warfarin and alcohol is complex. For occasional drinkers, alcohol may increase the bleeding risk associated with warfarin (alcohol increases warfarin's effects). Usually one or two drinks two to three times a week will not cause serious problems. In chronic drinkers (more than three drinks a day), alcohol causes more serious interactions with warfarin and decreases its effectiveness.[9] If you drink regularly, consult with your physician about whether you should stop altogether while you are taking warfarin (see Table 10.2).

It has been recommended that drinking alcohol and taking any nonsteroidal anti-inflammatory drug (e.g., ibuprofen, naproxen) should be separated by at least twelve hours. For a person drinking more than three drinks a day, these drugs should not be taken without a physician's approval because the combination increases the risk of gastric bleeding and ulcers. Such interactions may be severe enough to require hospitalization.[10]

Smoking and Your Medications

Approximately 4,800 compounds, including nicotine, are found in tobacco smoke. Smoking can induce metabolism of several drugs by the liver, causing treatment failure. Interestingly, it is cigarette smoke, not nicotine, that is responsible for pharmacokinetic drug interactions. Therefore, nicotine replacement therapy does not cause any drug interaction.[11] Theophylline, which is used in treating patients with asthma, is metabolized by the liver enzymes, and in smokers, blood levels of this drug can be reduced as much as 50 percent, causing treatment failure. Decreased blood levels of other drugs such as caffeine, chlorpromazine, clozapine, flecainide, fluvoxamine, haloperidol, mexiletine, olanzapine, propranolol, and tacrine may also be observed in patients who smoke regularly. Smokers may need a higher dosage of a sleeping aid (e.g., valium, alprazolam) for response and may require higher amounts of drugs (codeine, propoxyphene) for pain relief. In general, smokers may require higher doses than nonsmokers in order to achieve clinical responses.[12] Warfarin disposition in smokers is also reduced compared with that in nonsmokers, reducing the drug's efficacy.[13]

Possible Drug Interactions with Grapefruit Juice

The first interaction between grapefruit juice and a drug was reported in 1991. Bailey et al. found that a single glass of grapefruit juice caused a two- to threefold increase in the plasma concentration of felodipine, a calcium channel blocker, after oral intake of a 5 mg tablet; however, a similar amount of orange juice showed no effect.[14] Many subsequent investigations demonstrated that approximately forty other drugs have similar clinically important interactions with grapefruit juice.[15] Drinking grapefruit juice increases blood concentrations of many drugs due to increased absorption from the gut, and increased blood concentrations of these drugs may lead to adverse effects. Interestingly, few drugs show reduced blood concentrations due to the interaction with grapefruit juice, and a number of drugs show no interaction at all. Moreover, interaction of grapefruit juice with a drug is observed only if the drug is taken orally; no interaction is observed if the same drug is given by intramuscular or intravenous injection.

The cytochrome P-450 (CYP-450) family of enzymes, which are responsible for the metabolism of approximately 60 percent of all drugs by the liver, are also found in the small intestine. These enzymes break down drugs after oral intake. In addition, P-glycoproteins are also found in the gut. P-glycoproteins are part of a large family of efflux transporters, which are also found in the gonads, kidneys, brain, biliary system, and other organs. These proteins protect the body from harmful substances. In the kidneys, these proteins put drugs into the urine, but they pump the drug out of the brain.

Although grapefruit juice has many beneficial components and is also high in vitamin C, some of its components inhibit the action of the CYP enzymes in the small intestine and P-glycoprotein action in the gut. Therefore, breakdown of drugs in the small intestine is inhibited and more drugs enter into the bloodstream. In addition, due to blocked action of P-glycoprotein, drugs already absorbed are not pumped back into the gut, and their concentration in the bloodstream is significantly increased.[16] Furanocoumarins found in grapefruit juice are probably responsible for these interactions. The major furanocoumarin in grapefruit juice is bergamottin, which inhibits CYP-450 in tests performed *in vitro* (outside the body).[17] Furanocoumarin-containing drinks such as Sun Drop citrus soda may also produce grapefruit juice-like effects, but furanocoumarin-free grapefruit juice does not interact with any drugs.[18]

Drinking only one glass of grapefruit juice (200–250 mL) is sufficient to produce interaction with certain drugs.[19] Eating a whole grapefruit may also produce such interaction, though the time of ingestion is also important. While most of the effects of grapefruit juice last up to twelve hours after ingestion, some reports indicate that they may last as long as twenty-four hours.

Table 10.3 identifies various drugs that interact with grapefruit juice.

TABLE 10.3: Grapefruit Juice–Drug Interactions

CLASS OF MEDICATION	DRUG	EFFECT
Antianxiety drugs	Diazepam, midazolam, triazolam, buspirone, alprazolam (no interaction)	Increased blood level, which may cause dizziness, drowsiness, and poor motor function
Anticoagulants	Warfarin	Controversies in literature: no effect/increased effect of warfarin
Anticonvulsants	Carbamazepine, phenytoin (no interaction)	Increased blood level/adverse effect
Antihistamines	Terfenadine, fexofenadine (lower blood level/no effect)	Increased blood level/cardiac toxicity
Calcium channel blockers (anti-hypertensives)	Felodipine, nitrendipine, nisoldipine, nimodipine, pranidipine, nicardipine, verapamil, nifedipine (no interaction), amiodarone (no interaction), diltiazem (no interaction)	Increased blood level, which may cause low blood pressure and irregular heartbeat
Cardioactive drugs	Amiodarone, digoxin (no interaction)	Blocked metabolism/cardiac toxicity
Cholesterol-lowering drugs	Atorvastatin, lovastatin, simvastatin, pravastatin (no interaction)	Increased blood level, which may cause liver damage, rhabdomyolysis, and acute renal failure
Erectile-dysfunction drugs	Sildenafil	Increased blood level
Gastrointestinal-disorder drugs	Cisapride	Increased blood level/cardiac
Immuno-suppressants	Cyclosporine, tacrolimus (delayed interaction, which means the effects are seen some time after taking these drugs and grapefruit juice)	Increased blood level may cause kidney damage

The most significant interactions between grapefruit juice and drugs occur with drugs that block the calcium channel (calcium channel blockers are used to treat angina pectoris and hypertension); for example, felodipine. These drugs are used to treat hypertension and angina pectoris. Some, like felodipine, are poorly absorbed from the gut. But in the presence of grapefruit juice, significantly more drug is absorbed, resulting in a high concentration of felodipine in the blood. Other drugs in this class, for example, nicardipine, verapamil, and nimodipine, demonstrate similar interactions with grapefruit juice. On the other hand, drugs that are absorbed significantly from the gut, such as amlodipine and nifedipine, show no significant interaction with grapefruit juice. When the blood level of a calcium channel blocker is increased significantly due to the interaction with grapefruit juice, adverse effects of the drugs, such as hypotension and increased heart rate, are observed.[20]

If you are taking any medication for the treatment of a chronic condition (e.g., high blood pressure), please consult with your health-care provider about whether or not you should drink grapefruit juice on a regular basis.

The benzodiazepine family of drugs is widely prescribed worldwide as sedative-hypnotic agents for the treatment of anxiety and depression, and also to aid sleep. Certain drugs in this class—diazepam, midazolam, and triazolam—interact with grapefruit juice, significantly increasing levels of these drugs in the blood. Such interactions may cause increased sedation. However, another widely prescribed benzodiazepine medication, alprazolam (Xanax), demonstrated no interaction with grapefruit juice. A non-benzodiazepine sedative/hypnotic drug, buspirone, which is poorly absorbed from the gut, showed high blood concentration due to the interaction with grapefruit juice, causing toxicity.[21] Grapefruit juice should be avoided if you are taking buspirone.

Cholesterol-lowering drugs such as simvastatin, atorvastatin, and lovastatin show increased blood concentrations due to the interaction with grapefruit juice. However, the cholesterol-lowering drug pravastatin demonstrated no interaction with grapefruit juice. If you are taking simvastatin, atorvastatin, or lovastatin, it is wise not to drink grapefruit juice because increased blood concentrations of these drugs may cause liver problems or even rhabdomyolysis (acute breakdown of skeletal muscle, causing release of myoglobin in the blood, which may cause renal failure) and acute renal failure.[22]

Grapefruit juice increases the blood level of cyclosporine, an immunosuppressant given to transplant recipients to prevent organ rejection, but no effect is observed if cyclosporine is administered intravenously. Increased cyclosporine concentration in the blood may cause damage to the kidneys, so you should avoid grapefruit juice if you are taking this drug.[23]

CASE STUDY

Sun Drop citrus soda caused interaction with cyclosporine in a thirty-two-year-old transplant recipient; cyclosporine concentration in the blood was increased by over 100 percent. The patient was drinking the soda, which contains furocoumarine, for breakfast.[24] Delayed effect of grapefruit juice on the blood level of tacrolimus, another immunosuppressant drug, has been reported in a liver transplant recipient. The patient demonstrated a considerable increase in trough blood concentration (blood level of tacrolimus prior to the next dose) of tacrolimus after ingestion of grapefruit juice (250 mL) four times a day for three days. The trough blood concentrations were not affected during or immediately after repeated intake of grapefruit juice. However, almost one week after ingestion of grapefruit juice, the blood tacrolimus concentration in this patient increased almost tenfold, thus increasing the potential for adverse effects from the drug.[25]

Grapefruit juice increases the blood concentration of carbamazepine, a drug used in treating epilepsy, by almost 100 percent, according to a published report.[26] However, no interaction was observed between grapefruit juice and phenytoin, which is also used in treating patients with epilepsy.[27] The blood concentration of sildenafil (Viagra), used to treat erectile dysfunction, is also increased due to the interaction with grapefruit juice. You should avoid drinking grapefruit juice when taking this drug.[28] In the presence of grapefruit juice, cisapride, used in treating gastrointestinal disorders, has shown increased blood concentration by as much as 50 percent, thus increasing the possibility of an adverse effects, including serious cardiac effects, from this drug.[29]

Combining terfenadine (used for treating allergies) and grapefruit juice may cause death.

CASE STUDY

A twenty-nine-year-old man who was taking terfenadine twice daily for more than a year collapsed and died when he consumed two glasses of grapefruit juice. His blood level of terfenadine was very high, and the coroner concluded that the death was due to cardiac arrest caused by terfenadine toxicity.[30]

Due to its cardiac toxicity, terfenadine has now been superseded by fexo-fenadine. Interestingly, grapefruit juice decreases the blood level of fexofenadine through a complex mechanism.[31]

Saquinavir, an HIV protease inhibitor used in treating patients with AIDS, is poorly absorbed from the gut, but in the presence of 400 mL (~1¾ cups) of grapefruit juice, absorption is significantly increased. This effect was absent when saquinavir was administered intravenously.[32] In contrast, grapefruit juice slightly decreased the blood level of another HIV protease inhibitor, amprenavir.[33] Grapefruit juice showed no interaction with indinavir, which belongs to the same class of drugs.[34]

Several drugs, such as alprazolam, digoxin, diltiazem, nifedipine, pravastatin, and haloperidol, have no reported interaction with grapefruit juice.[35] Other drugs, such as itraconazole, have minimal interaction.

Drug Interactions with Orange Juice

The sweet orange juice (regular orange juice) consumed throughout most of the world does not contain any furanocoumarin, and therefore few drug interactions with orange juice have been reported. On the other hand, the sour orange, also known as bitter or Seville orange, is different from a sweet orange. Seville orange juice contains furanocoumarin and may behave similarly to grapefruit juice when it interacts with various drugs. Malhotra et al. reported that Seville orange juice increased the blood level of felodipine with a mechanism similar to that of grapefruit juice.[36] Orange juice substantially reduced the absorption of celiprolol, a beta-blocking agent used in the treatment of hypertension, and therefore efficacy of the drug may be substantially reduced if taken after drinking orange juice. In a study involving ten healthy volunteers who drank 200 mL of orange juice, blood levels of celiprolol were reduced by approximately 89 percent.[37] Another report indicated that orange juice reduced the blood level of clofazimine (used in the treatment of multi-drug-resistant tuberculosis and leprosy).[38]

On the other hand, orange juice increased the absorption of the cholesterol-lowering drug pravastatin in healthy volunteers when the drug was administered orally, but it had no effect on the absorption of simvastatin.[39] Interestingly, grapefruit juice shows no interaction with pravastatin. Orange juice also enhances aluminum absorption from antacid preparations.

Drug Interactions with Pomelo, Cranberry, and Pomegranate Juices

Pomelo is closely related to grapefruit, and pomelo juice also contains various furanocoumarins. Therefore, the type of drug interaction associated with grapefruit juice is also possible after drinking pomelo juice. Increased blood concentrations of the immunosuppressant drugs cyclosporine and tacrolimus due to the interaction with pomelo juice have been reported.[40]

Although cranberry juice can also inhibit CYP-450, it does not interact with cyclosporine.[41] However, the interaction between cranberry juice and warfarin (used for preventing blood clots) is clinically very significant and may be fatal.

> After a chest infection, a man had a poor appetite and consumed nothing but cranberry juice for two weeks. He was also taking his regular drugs (digoxin, phenytoin, and warfarin). Six weeks after starting with cranberry juice he was admitted to the hospital with severe bleeding and died of internal bleeding (gastrointestinal and pericardial hemorrhage). Cranberry juice contains flavonoids that can inhibit enzymes that metabolize warfarin. Therefore, high blood levels of warfarin caused death to this person.[42]

CASE STUDY

Other cases of bleeding problems due to the interaction of warfarin with cranberry juice have been reported.

> *If you are taking warfarin, you should never drink cranberry juice.*

Pomegranate juice, like grapefruit juice, can inhibit intestinal CYP-450, thus causing drug interactions similar to those caused by grapefruit juice.

> A forty-eight-year-old man was taking 10 mg of ezetimibe a day and 5 mg of rosuvastatin every other day to lower his cholesterol. Three weeks before being admitted to the hospital with severe thigh pain, general malaise, and brown urine, he started drinking pomegranate juice after reading a report about its health benefits. He was diagnosed with rhabdomyolysis. The concentration marker of skeletal muscle damage, creatinine kinase, was very high in his blood. Because rhabdomyolysis is a serious side effect of cholesterol-lowering drugs due to high

CASE STUDY

blood concentrations, he was told to stop taking the medications and pomegranate juice, and his disease was resolved in a few days.[43]

Therefore, pomegranate juice, like grapefruit juice, may increase the blood concentrations of many drugs including felodipine, nicardipine, nimodipine, lovastatin, simvastatin, atorvastatin, cyclosporine, and saquinavir. Consult your physician before drinking pomegranate juice if you are taking any medication for treating a chronic disease.

Conclusion

Food-drug interactions can have clinical significance. Eating an excess amount of vegetables that are high in vitamin K may significantly reduce the efficacy of warfarin. Mixing alcohol with certain drugs is dangerous. Grapefruit juice contains furocoumarin, which inhibits intestinal CYP-450 and increases the absorption of many drugs from the gut. Therefore, patients drinking grapefruit juice and taking such medications are at a higher risk of having adverse effects. Please consult with your doctor to determine whether drinking grapefruit juice is safe for you. If you are taking warfarin, you should also avoid cranberry juice. Pomegranate juice can also inhibit CYP-450 in the intestine, causing interactions with various drugs.

CHAPTER 11

Herbal Supplements, Alternative Therapies, and Women's Health

In general, women use complementary and alternative therapies, including taking herbal supplements, more than men. Many women use herbal products and alternative therapies such as aromatherapy massage, acupressure, acupunture, hyponosis, etc., when going through menopause. In addition, women use herbs to improve their general well-being and reproductive health, and to reduce the discomfort of the menstrual cycle. Women also take heral supplements during pregnancy (extreme care must be taken to select safe herbal supplements during pregnancy because many supplements can harm the fetus and/or may cause miscarriage). This chapter discusses the herbal supplements and alternative therapies used more frequently by women or exclusively by women, as well as their safety and efficacy.

Supplements and Remedies Used at Menopause

One common reason for a woman to use an herbal supplement or alternative therapy is for relief from symptoms of menopause. Approximately two-thirds of women who reach menopause experience menopausal symptoms, especially hot flashes. For a long time, hormone-replacement therapy was considered a solution for these symptoms, but given the controversies regarding its potential dangers, particularly the increased risk of developing cancer, many women turn to herbal supplements and other complementary and alternative therapies instead. Perimenopausal and postmenopausal women are the biggest users of herbal supplements, and 70 percent of women do not tell their health-care provider that they use alternative therapies. Among the herbal supplements used for relief of menopausal symptoms are black cohosh, soy, red clover, chasteberry, hops, evening primrose, Dong Quai, ginkgo, ginseng, kava, valerian, licorice root, motherwort, St. John's wort, lemon balm, and wild yam. Scientific evidence to date suggests that black cohosh is safe and effective for reducing menopausal symptoms, especially hot flashes and mood swings. Products containing plant estrogens (phytoestrogens), such as soy and red clover, may have some effect, and these supplements also have other positive health effects such as reducing lipids and the risk of heart attack. St. John's wort is effective in treating mood swings related to menopausal transition. There is limited evidence regarding the safety and efficacy of some other herbal supplements taken for treating menopausal symptoms.[1]

Supplements and Remedies Used During Pregnancy

Pregnant women use complementary and alternative therapies including herbal supplements in order to find relief from the discomforts of pregnancy. A survey of two hundred women in the United States showed that 15 percent use herbal supplements, most commonly ginger, vitamin B$_6$, chamomile, and cola (the nut, not the soda). Another survey indicates that the most commonly used herbal supplements during pregnancy are garlic, aloe, chamomile, peppermint, ginger, echinacea, pumpkin seed, and ginseng.

More interesting, a survey of five hundred members of the American College of Nurse-Midwives indicated that more than half of them employed herbal supplements for inducing labor. The herbal supplements most commonly used were blue cohosh, black cohosh, red raspberry leaves, castor oil, and Evening-primrose oil. Currently, there is no compelling scientific evidence that these supplements are effective in inducing labor.[2]

Pregnant women should be extremely careful in using herbal supplements because many may induce miscarriage. Moreover, some may harm the fetus. Similarly, nursing mothers should be aware that components of herbal supplements may be secreted in breast milk and harm the newborn. Researchers Marcus and Snodgrass recommended that pregnant women avoid all herbal supplements in order to be on the safe side.[3]

It is true that many over-the-counter medicines should also be avoided during pregnancy and some may cause birth defects; for example, the use of the antibiotic tetracycline during pregnancy causes the baby's teeth to have yellow stains. However, doctors are well aware of such ill effects of certain medicines and do not prescribe them for pregnant women. Many Western medicines that should be avoided during pregnancy can be used safely by women who are not pregnant. Currently, the safety of only a few herbal supplements has been established for use during pregnancy. However, certain herbal supplements that are fairly safe normally may cause adverse reactions during pregnancy. For example, black cohosh is safe and effective in treating symptoms of menopause, but it should be avoided by pregnant women because it may cause miscarriage.

Professor Edzard Ernst of the Department of Complementary Medicine, School of Sports and Health Sciences, at the University of Exeter in the United Kingdom compiled a long list of herbal supplements that should be avoided during pregnancy.[4] The following herbal remedies, taken from that list, are those most commonly used in the United States:

Herbal Remedies That Should Be Avoided During Pregnancy

- alfalfa
- aloe vera
- ashwagandha
- barberry
- basil
- bearberry
- bitter lemon
- black cohosh
- blue cohosh
- borage
- broom
- buckthorn
- bugleweed
- burdock
- buttercup
- calamus
- calendula
- camphor
- cascara sagrada
- castor bean
- catnip
- celandine
- celery
- chamomile
- chaste tree
- cinnamon
- cola
- coltsfoot
- comfrey
- cotton-root bark
- Dong Quai
- ephedra (Ma Huang)
- fennel
- feverfew
- flaxseed
- goldenseal
- hyssop
- juniper
- kava
- lavender
- licorice
- lobelia
- mistletoe
- motherwort
- oregano
- parsley
- passionflower
- pennyroyal
- periwinkle
- saffron
- sage
- St. John's wort
- sandalwood
- sassafras
- senna
- skullcap
- slippery elm
- sticky nightshade
- tansy
- valerian
- wild cherry
- wild ginger
- wormseed
- wormwood
- yellow cedar
- yohimbe

In my opinion, if you are pregnant, you should avoid all herbal supplements if possible. If you really want to use one or two relatively safe supplements during pregnancy, please do not take them without permission from your doctor.

During pregnancy, you may wish to consider alternative therapies such as aromatherapy massage, acupressure massage, acupuncture, Reiki, and energy work for beneficial effects without any danger of harm. After childbirth, acupuncture and aromatherapy massage can be helpful in treating postpartum depression. The benefits of these alternative therapies are discussed later in this chapter.

Dangerous Herbs During Pregnancy

Although certain herbal supplements listed above have borderline toxicity during pregnancy, others may cause miscarriage or other serious side effects and must not be taken. Agnus castus is a popular British herbal remedy that is indicated for maintaining a healthy menstrual cycle and relieving symptoms of menopause. This herb has estrogen-like activity and may cause ovarian stimulation, leading to miscarriage. Blue cohosh is used in pregnancy and lactation and also for inducing labor. One woman took blue cohosh to promote uterine contraction for delivery. The infant suffered heart attack and cardiac shock and was critically ill for several weeks. The cardiotoxic compounds found in blue cohosh may be responsible for these serious toxic effects on the newborn. Blue cohosh also has abortifacient properties and may have the potential to cause damage to a fetus.[5] Chamomile, the Chinese medicine Dong Quai, fennel, goldenseal, and passionflower can cause miscarriage and should be avoided during pregnancy. Pine and juniper contain high amounts of isocupressic acid and also have abortifacient effects.[6] Black cohosh has labor-inducing properties and may cause miscarriage.[7]

In one report, the authors commented that several herbal supplements are indeed intended for causing abortion and may be effective in doing so. These include parsley, cola de quirquincho, the South American herbal proprietary remedy Carachipita (which contains pennyroyal), fennel, celery, and other, less-common herbal supplements.[8]

It should be noted that even the alcohol content of an herbal remedy can hurt a fetus.

There was a report of fetal alcohol syndrome (permanent birth defects due to the fetus's exposure to alcohol) that was associated with the use of an herbal tonic by a twenty-nine-year-old Chinese woman during her pregnancy. The herbal preparation was 19 percent alcohol, and the mother took this supplement early in her pregnancy.[9]

The following is a list of common herbs that may cause miscarriage:

Common Herbs That May Cause Miscarriage

- blue cohosh
- burdock
- chamomile
- Dong Quai
- flaxseed
- juniper
- parsley
- pennyroyal
- saffron
- sticky nightshade
- black cohosh
- celery
- cotton root bark
- fennel
- goldenseal
- Ma Huang
- passionflower
- periwinkle
- slippery elm
- tansy

Relatively Safe Herbs in Pregnancy

There are few relatively safe herbs that can be safely used during pregnancy. Echinacea is one. In a Canadian study involving 412 pregnant women (206 women took echinacea and 206 women did not), there was no major difference in observed birth defects between the two groups. There were 195 live births in the echinacea group and 198 live births in the control group, with 13 spontaneous abortions in the echinacea group and 7 spontaneous abortions in the control group. There was no statistical difference between the echinacea group and the control group in outcome of pregnancy. This study suggests that use of echinacea is not associated with an increased risk of birth defects in pregnancy.[10]

Cranberry is effective in treating urinary tract infection, which is good news for pregnant women, since they experience urinary tract infection with greater frequency during pregnancy. There is no direct evidence of either safety or harm to mother or fetus as a result of consuming cranberry during pregnancy. Therefore, cranberry fruit or juice may be a valuable therapeutic choice for treating urinary tract infections during pregnancy.[11]

One recent study using 70 women concluded that ginger is more effective than vitamin B_6 in reducing the severity of nausea and is equally as effective as vitamin B_6 for decreasing the number of vomiting episodes during early pregnancy.[12] In another study the authors analyzed data from six clinical trials involving 675 pregnant women and one cohort study involving 187 subjects and concluded that ginger was as effective as vitamin B_6 in relieving nausea and reducing vomiting episodes in pregnant women. Follow-up studies showed no adverse effect of ginger on the outcome of pregnancy.[13]

Herbs That Are Effective in Treating Other Women's Health Issues

Several herbal supplements that are unsafe for use during pregnancy are safe and effective in treating various women's health issues. Herbal supplements such as black cohosh, soy, and red clover are effective in relieving symptoms of menopause. Others are effective in treating premenstrual symptoms.

Black Cohosh

Black cohosh, a native North American plant, has been used by Native Americans to treat various conditions in women, including menopausal symptoms. Clinical studies in Germany have shown that black cohosh is effective in relieving symptoms of menopause, including hot flashes and mood swings. The German health authorities approved the use of black cohosh (Remifemin brand), at 40 mg a day for six months, for menopausal symptoms. Black cohosh has a good safety record if used for six months or less. However, there are a few case reports of severe liver toxicity from the use of black cohosh, although the toxicity cannot be established as solely due to the black cohosh.

> *Due to suspected liver toxicity from black cohosh, you should inform your doctor if you are using it so that appropriate blood tests can be ordered to ensure that you are not experiencing liver toxicity.*

Although earlier research papers reported that black cohosh has estrogen-like effects, recent findings have shown that it is not estrogenic. In summary, black cohosh is an effective herbal supplement for relieving menopausal symptoms except for a few reports of liver toxicity (see also Chapter 7). In addition, black cohosh should not be used for more than six months because long-term safety has not been established. Pregnant women and lactating mothers should not take black cohosh under any circumstances.

Chaste Tree (Chasteberry)

Extract of the fruits (berries) of the chaste tree (*Vitex agnus-castus*) is widely used in treating premenstrual symptoms and irregularities in the menstrual cycle, and to stimulate breast-milk production. Scientific studies have shown that chasteberry extracts are beneficial in treating the most common premenstrual symptom, premenstrual breast pain (mastalgia, or mastodynia). In mastalgia, women release more prolactin, a hormone. Studies have shown that chasteberry extract can reduce such high prolactin levels in the blood, thus providing relief.[14]

Essential oil extracted from both chasteberry and chaste-tree leaves was also found to be effective in relieving symptoms of menopause.[15] Chasteberry extract is a safe and effective herbal supplement. Data from clinical trials, post-marketing surveillance studies, surveys, spontaneous reporting schemes, manufacturers, and herbalists indicate that adverse events following the use of chasteberry extracts are mild and reversible. The most common side effects are nausea, gastrointestinal disturbances, menstrual disorders, acne, itchiness, and rash. However, chasteberry extract should be avoided during pregnancy and during lactation.[16]

Cranberry

Native Americans used cranberry as a food, a dye, and a medicine. Cranberry juice is widely taken for symptomatic relief of urinary tract infection. It is also given to help reduce urinary odor. It is believed that cranberry juice can decrease the rate of formation of kidney stones. Cranberry is available as powder in capsules, as well as in juice and sauce form.

Approximately 60 percent of women experience a urinary tract infection (UTI) during their lifetimes, and for many it is a recurring problem. Cranberry juice is an effective treatment for symptomatic relief of a UTI. In one study, the authors reviewed data from nine clinical trials and concluded that over twelve months, cranberry products significantly reduced the incidence of UTI, particularly in women with recurrent infections.[17] In another study, forty-seven subjects with spinal-cord injury and documented neurogenic bladder (in which patients have difficulty passing urine) received cranberry tablets for one month for preventing UTI, followed by an alternate preparation for an additional six months. During the study period, the subjects who were taking cranberry had seven UTIs, compared with subjects taking a placebo (instead of cranberry), who had twenty-one UTIs. The authors concluded that cranberry extract tablets should be considered for the prevention of UTIs in spinal-cord-injury patients with a neurogenic bladder.[18] In a recent article, researchers concluded that the antibiotic trimethoprim had very little advantage over cranberry extract in the prevention of recurrent UTIs in older women. Moreover, the antibiotic has more adverse effects than cranberry.[19] Cranberry extract may also have activity against *H. pylori* bacteria (responsible for the majority of peptic ulcers) and is effective in lowering total cholesterol and LDL ("bad") cholesterol in diabetic patients.[20]

Dong Quai

Dong Quai is the popular name of *Angelica sinensis*, a tall, white-flowered plant that grows in China, Japan, and Korea. The dried root has medicinal values and has been traditionally used in China for treating abnormal menstruation and menopausal symptoms. Dong Quai is also considered a female tonic. This herb has several pharmacological properties, including anticoagulation and antiplatelet activity (blood thinner). It may also support the immune system. Dong Quai is most commonly used in the United States for the relief of menopausal symptoms, including hot flashes, skin flushing, perspiration, and chills.

Used alone, Dong Quai has very little effect in relieving symptoms of menopause, and traditional Chinese herbalists never prescribe it as a single supplement. In one clinical trial involving seventy-one postmenopausal women who used Dong Quai for twenty-four weeks, no beneficial effect was observed in preventing symptoms. Dong Quai does not contain any significant amount of phytoestrogen. However, in combination with other herbs Dong Quai may produce beneficial effects in reducing symptoms of menopause.[21] In a recently published article, the authors commented that the Chinese herbal preparation Dang Gui Bu Xue Tang, which contains both Dong Quai and astragalus, is effective in reducing mild hot flashes in postmenopausal women but not in reducing the frequency of moderate to severe hot flashes.[22] Note that Dong Quai interacts with anticoagulation therapy involving warfarin (see Chapter 10).

Hops

Hops (*Humulus lupulus*) is a climbing perennial vine native to Europe that can also be found in North America, Asia, and Australia. The female flowers that mature in the summer have been used traditionally as a food additive in beer in order to give it its bitter taste and aroma. Hops extracts are considered generally safe for human consumption and are on the FDA GRAS list. Traditionally, hops extracts were used as sedatives and also to control mania and other symptoms. However, hops is rich in phytoestrogen, including 8-prenylnaringenin (8-PN), which is known to interact weakly with estrogen receptors and may be effective for relieving symptoms of menopause. One clinical trial involving sixty-seven menopausal women over a period of twelve weeks demonstrated that hops extract standardized for 8-PN was effective in reducing the discomforts of menopause. The authors concluded that daily intake of hops extract standardized to 8-PN as a potent phytoestrogen exerted favorable effects in alleviating menopausal symptoms, including hot flashes, and is a good alternative treatment.[23]

Red Clover

Red clover is a native North American plant that has traditionally been used as an anticancer and an antispasmodic agent. However, it also contains several isoflavones, which act as phytoestrogens. The use of red clover for treating menopausal symptoms is fairly recent. Clinical trials evaluating its efficacy produced mixed results. In two studies where the subjects took red-clover supplements for up to twelve weeks, no significant improvement in symptoms was observed in the women who took red clover versus women who took a placebo. In contrast, two other studies found statistically significant reductions in hot flashes in women who took red-clover supplement. Generally, it is believed that isoflavone and coumestan are the components responsible for red clover's estrogen-like effect. One of the most commonly used red-clover products is Promensil, a red-clover derivative with concentrated levels of isoflavones.[24]

Red clover is also suggested as a treatment for osteoporosis. In one study, women who took red-clover supplement lost less bone mineral density (BMD) than the group that did not take red clover. Another study reported that women in the red-clover group had improved BMD. Although three trials did not show any beneficial effect of red clover in improving lipid profile, one clinical study showed that red-clover extract significantly improved the concentration of "good" (HDL) cholesterol in postmenopausal women. In this study, the authors recruited forty-six postmenopausal women and gave them either a red-clover, isoflavone preparation (Rimostil) containing genistein, daidzein, formononetin, and biochanin, or a placebo. After six months, HDL was significantly increased (15.7–28.6 percent) in women who took the red-clover supplement, and the increases did not depend on the dose. In addition, these women also showed significant increases in bone density.[25] No adverse effects of red-clover leaf extracts have been reported in clinical trials and in the medical literature, but most studies conducted using red clover lasted only six to twelve months. At this point, the safety of red-clover extract in pregnant and lactating mothers and in women who have breast cancer or hormone-sensitive cancer has not been established.

Soy

There is much current interest in using soy foods for treating menopausal symptoms because soy contains phytoestrogens such as formononetin, biochanin A, daidzein, and genistein. These compounds are also present in red-clover extract because both plants belong to the same family (legumes). Asian diets are high in soy protein, and many women in these countries experience few menopausal complaints. However, it is not completely understood whether the lower prevalence of hot flashes and other menopausal symptoms is due to a soy diet or a combination of diet and cultural factors. The scientific research showed that soy has a protective effect on breast and endometrial cancer. Case-controlled studies in Asian countries demonstrate decreased rates of breast cancer. However, when the Japanese women moved to the United States, their risk for cancer increased.[26]

Clinical trials evaluating the efficacy of soy supplements in alleviating menopausal symptoms showed mixed results. Some large clinical trials failed to show any beneficial effect of soy in relieving symptoms of menopause, while others showed marginal to significant efficacy. In one study, women experienced significant reductions in incidence of hot flashes after six weeks of taking soy supplements (400 mg/day), compared with those taking the placebo.[27] In a recent clinical trial involving eighty postmenopausal women who received a soy supplement (250 mg soy extract), isoflavone (100 mg), or a placebo, the authors observed that after ten months there was a significant reduction in hot flashes among isoflavone and soy supplement users compared with the placebo group. Moreover, isoflavone, in combination with soy extract, was significantly superior to soy extract alone in reducing hot-flash severity. No serious adverse effect was observed in any women in this study. The authors concluded that soy isoflavone extract has favorable effects on relieving symptoms of menopause and is a safe and effective alternative therapy for postmenopausal women.[28]

Soy is also effective in improving bone mineral density (BMD) in postmenopausal women and thus may help prevent osteoporosis. Clinical studies in general showed a beneficial effect of soy supplements in bone mineral density, bone-turnover markers, and bone mechanical strength in postmenopausal women.[29] In addition, soy has a favorable effect on lipid profile and reduces total cholesterol and "bad" (LDL) cholesterol while increasing "good" (HDL) cholesterol. Although soy contains phytoestrogens, clinical studies indicate that it does not increase the risk of breast cancer. Soy extracts are well tolerated, with few reported side effects. Unless you have a soy allergy, you can safely consume soy foods.

Herbs That Are Not Effective or for Which There Is Insufficient Data

Many other herbs are used for various women's health issues, but in general these supplements are ineffective or there is not enough data to reach a conclusion regarding their safety and efficacy. The most commonly used herbs in this category are discussed below. In addition, women also take many other herbal supplements such as valerian, ginkgo, St. John's wort, and ginseng, which are discussed in depth in Chapter 2.

Evening-Primrose Oil

Evening-primrose oil is extracted from the seed of the evening primrose, a native North American flowering plant, and this oil is rich in essential fatty acids such as linoleic acid and gamma-linolenic acid. Although evening-primrose oil offers other health benefits, clinical trials have failed to show any effects in relieving symptoms of menopause. Evening-primrose oil is usually well tolerated, and side effects, such as nausea, diarrhea, and bloating, are mild.[30]

Mexican, or Wild, Yam

Wild yam, also known as Mexican yam, is a perennial vine whose root is referred to as "colic root" because it has been traditionally used for treating gastrointestinal irritation and spasm. In folk medicine, wild yam has been used for treating menstrual cramps and postpartum pain. Despite popular claims and promotion, limited scientific research at this point has failed to show any significant benefit of wild yam for relieving symptoms of menopause because its estrogen-like compounds are not active in the human body.[31] In one study, the authors evaluated the efficacy of wild-yam cream in twenty-three women suffering from symptoms of menopause and concluded that short-term use of topical wild-yam extract is free from side effects but appears to have little effect on menopausal symptoms.[32]

Motherwort

Motherwort is a flowering plant of the mint family with a long history of medicinal use because of its perceived calming effect on the heart and especially for stopping palpitations. It is found in herbal supplements either alone or in combination with black cohosh for treating symptoms of menopause, but at this point scientific data regarding its safety and efficacy is lacking. However, data from a clinical trial involving 301 women showed that black cohosh in combination with the herbal antidepressant St. John's wort is effective in treating symptoms of menopause, including hot flashes, irritability, minor depression, mood swings, and insomnia.[33]

Raspberry Leaf Extract

Raspberry bushes are native to North America and are known for their delicious red berries (*Rubus idaeus*), but raspberry leaves have long been used in traditional folk medicine for treating diarrhea, sore throat, and colds as well as for pregnancy and postpartum support. It is believed that red-raspberry leaf extract can act as a uterine relaxant and be used to shorten the time of labor. Scientific research has demonstrated that red-raspberry leaf extract has antioxidant, antibacterial, and anti-infective properties and also can be effective in relieving pain and anxiety.[34] Parson et al., studying 108 women (57 consumed raspberry leaf product, and 51 did not), observed that consumption of raspberry leaf extract shortened the time of labor. In addition, women who consumed raspberry leaf extract were also less likely to suffer artificial rupture of their membranes or require a cesarean section, forceps, or vacuum birth than women who did not take raspberry leaf extract.[35] However, Simpson et al. reported in an article that although raspberry leaf consumed in tablet form caused no adverse effect to the mother or baby, and raspberry leaf product did not shorten the first stage of labor, it did seem to shorten the second stage of labor and lead to a lower rate of forceps deliveries.[36]

Aromatherapy, Acupuncture, and Acupressure

Acupuncture may be effective in reducing the severity of hot flashes in menopausal women. Nir et al. conducted a pilot study using twenty-nine postmenopausal women who had at least seven moderate to severe hot flashes every day and observed that women who received active acupuncture treatment had a greater reduction in severity of hot flashes compared with women who received placebo treatment.[37] In another study, the authors concluded that aromatherapy massage could be effective in reducing symptoms of menopause.[38] Smith et al. reviewed data from three clinical trials (496 women) involving acupuncture, two trials with acupressure (172 women), one trial with aromatherapy (22 women), five trials with hypnosis (729 women), one trial with relaxation (34 women), and one trial with massage (60 women) and concluded that both acupuncture and hypnosis may be beneficial for the management of pain during labor. Women who taught themselves self-hypnosis and women who received acupuncture required less analgesic medicine for pain control during labor.[39] A recent report showed that acupressure application in pregnant women suffering from nausea and vomiting is effective in symptom control.[40]

Conclusion

Although many herbal supplements are promoted for relieving the symptoms of menopause, at this point only black cohosh, soy, and red clover have been proven in scientific studies to be effective in reducing the symptoms of menopause. In addition to herbal supplements, many other alternative therapies, such as aromatherapy, massage, acupressure, and acupuncture, may be effective in reducing menopausal symptoms. Cranberry is effective in treating urinary tract infections. However, pregnant women should be extremely careful before using any herbal supplement because the long-term safety profiles of many herbal supplements are not yet known. In addition, certain herbal supplements may cause miscarriage. Women who teach themselves self-hypnosis may require less pain medication during labor and delivery.

CHAPTER 12

How Herbal Remedies May Affect Laboratory Test Results

This chapter discusses which herbal remedies tend to alter test results and how they do so. Certain herbal supplements and traditional Chinese medicines may alter your laboratory test results. Because many patients do not tell their doctors that they are using herbal supplements, these unexpected test results may confuse their doctors. In one pilot study, the authors found that 62.5 percent of participants who used herbal supplements also used medications, but only 33 percent of these subjects reported their use of herbal supplements to their doctors. Only 3 percent of participants received information regarding herbal supplements from their doctors, nurses, or pharmacists. The majority of participants received information regarding their selection of herbal supplements from staff in health-food stores.[1]

An herbal remedy can affect laboratory test results by one of the three following mechanisms:

1. Physiological effects: When a remedy alters your body's normal physiology, changes in blood concentrations of certain chemicals may be observed. In addition, if an herbal remedy causes any organ damage, concentration of a specific marker for that organ may be elevated in the blood. (A marker is a substance found in a large amount in an organ but in a very small amount in the blood. When an organ is damaged, this compound may be released into the blood and can be detected by a laboratory test).

2. A component of an herbal remedy may be mistaken for a drug by the antibody used in the immunoassay (a biochemical test that uses specific proteins called antibodies to measure the concentration of a substance—a

drug or another protein—in biological liquids like blood and urine) for that particular drug.

3. If an herbal remedy is contaminated with a heavy metal (lead, mercury, or arsenic) or a Western drug, the unexpected presence of that drug in the blood of the patient may confuse the doctor. In addition, heavy-metal toxicity may result from taking certain herbal supplements. This topic is discussed in detail in Chapter 13.

Liver-Function Tests

Common causes of elevated liver enzymes such as alanine transaminase (ALT), aspartate transaminase (AST), alkaline phosphatase (ALP), and gamma-glutamyl transpeptidase (GGT or GGTP) are liver damage due to hepatitis and other related viruses. Elevated bilirubin (a breakdown product of heme, the nonprotein part of hemoglobin that contains iron) concentration in serum is also an indicator of liver damage. GGT concentration is elevated in chronic drinkers. As we discussed earlier (see Chapter 7), certain herbal supplements can cause significant liver damage, and elevated concentrations of ALT, AST, and bilirubin can be observed in the serum of individuals taking such supplements. These test results could confuse the physician if the patient does not disclose the use of herbal supplements. Supplements that cause damage to the liver are discussed in detail in Chapter 7. In general, kava, chaparral, germander, mistletoe, pennyroyal oil, green-tea extract, noni juice, and a variety of other herbal supplements may cause abnormal liver-function tests in healthy individuals.

> A fifty-year-old man took three to four kava capsules daily for two months (maximum recommended dose is three capsules). Liver-function tests showed sixty- to seventyfold increases in AST and ALT. The patient eventually received a liver transplant.[2]
>
> **CASE STUDY**

> A forty-five-year-old man was admitted to the outpatient department with a two-week history of malaise, nausea, loss of appetite, fatigue, and nonspecific chest discomfort. He was not taking any medication. His liver enzymes, including LDH and GGT, were significantly elevated, although total bilirubin was normal. Based on the liver-function tests, he was diagnosed with acute viral hepatitis, but all
>
> **CASE STUDY**

blood tests for hepatitis were negative. The patient admitted to having drunk noni juice, a Polynesian remedy made from a tropical fruit, for three weeks prior to developing these symptoms. After he stopped drinking noni juice, his liver enzymes returned to normal values within one month.[3]

For a list of common herbal remedies that may cause abnormal liver-function tests, please see Chapter 7.

Glucose Tests

Carbohydrates play many essential roles in sustaining life, including storage and transport of energy. In plants, cellulose, a form of carbohydrate, is an essential component of the cell membrane. However, in the animal kingdom, cell membranes are composed of complex lipids, mainly phospholipids. The basic units of carbohydrates are various sugars (glucose, fructose, mannose, and galactose), or monosaccharides. The body metabolizes carbohydrates from food into glucose, a monosaccharide. Glucose is the primary source of energy in living organisms (both plants and animals). In humans, glucose is the primary fuel for the brain and muscles. Glucose is also called blood sugar because in healthy subjects it circulates in the blood at a concentration between 70 and 99 mg/dL (blood sugar or blood glucose is the concentration of glucose in serum); the concentration is expressed as mg per 100 mL of serum or mg per deciliter (mg/dL). The old guideline for normal blood sugar was 70–110 mg/dL, and some clinical laboratories still use this reference range for serum glucose level. Although the glucose in blood is loosely termed blood "sugar," table sugar is actually a disaccharide composed of one glucose molecule and one fructose molecule. Milk-sugar, or lactose, is composed of one glucose molecule and one galactose molecule. After intake these sugars are broken down by our body into simple monosaccharides.

Diabetes mellitus is a disease in which the body does not produce enough insulin (the hormone that converts sugar into energy), resulting in increased glucose concentrations in the blood. In type 1 diabetes, which is also called insulin-dependent diabetes, the production of insulin by the pancreas is minimal or zero, and insulin shots must be taken by these patients in order to maintain normal blood glucose levels. In patients with type 2 diabetes, also known as non-insulin-dependent diabetes, either insulin production is insufficient or, due to obesity or other factors, the insulin produced cannot be used properly by the muscle for breaking down glucose. This phenomenon is called insulin resistance. These patients can be treated with diet control, weight reduction, exercise, and medication, which may be taken orally. Some medications stimulate the pancreas to secrete more insulin, while other medications, such as metformin, help muscles to utilize insulin for breaking down sugar. Fasting blood glucose levels over 126 mg/dL may indicate onset of diabetes. Nonfasting blood sugar levels above 200 mg/dL or blood sugar levels above 200 mg/dL two hours after ingestion of 75 gm of glucose (glucose-tolerance test) may also indicate diabetes. In addition to type 1 and type 2 diabetes, there is also something called gestational diabetes, which afflicts some pregnant women.

Many herbal supplements such as ginseng, fenugreek, garlic, bitter melon, gymnema, psyllium, bilberry, dandelion, burdock, and prickly pear cactus can lower serum glucose levels. In addition, the dietary supplement chromium is capable of lowering serum glucose levels. Patients with diabetes should tightly maintain their serum glucose level through diet, exercise, and medication (oral drugs or insulin shots). Sometimes these patients take herbal supplements without approval of their doctors and experience lowered glucose levels (hypoglycemia). Hypoglycemia may cause many symptoms including dizziness, general weakness, and fatigue. Severe hypoglycemia (serum glucose less than 50 mg/dL) may cause the patient to faint and creates a medical emergency. Death may result from serum glucose levels less than 40 mg/dL. Although several herbal supplements and chromium show promise in controlling high glucose in the blood, a patient taking insulin or oral medication for diabetes should not take such supplements without consulting his or her physician because a lower amount of medication may be needed if such supplements are taken. Otherwise, these patients may suffer severe hypoglycemia requiring medical attention.

CASE STUDY

A forty-six-year-old woman was diagnosed with non-insulin-dependent diabetes, and her serum glucose was stabilized with diet, exercise, and glipizide. Ten months later she reported to the clinic following a three-day episode of low glucose levels ranging from 60 to 85 mg/dL on her home glucose-monitoring device. In the clinic, her non-fasting glucose (using a finger stick) was only 55 mg/dL. She was not taking any other medication, and there was no change in her lifestyle. The doctor treated her with glucagon to increase her serum glucose level, and when her glucose concentration reached 110 mg/dL, she felt much better.

At that point she admitted to having taken several herbal supplements: ginseng for lowering blood glucose and cholesterol, garlic to prevent heart disease, astragalus for lowering blood glucose, and juniper berry tea for digestion. These supplements were responsible for her abnormally low serum glucose and her symptoms.[4]

CASE STUDY

Mr. A. had been diagnosed with insulin-dependent diabetes mellitus at twenty years of age, and since that time he had been on insulin. His blood glucose ranged between 90 mg/dL and 120 mg/dL. One day at work after a long and physically strenuous shift, he became agitated and paranoid and started running around the office, falling and tripping, shouting and cursing at his coworkers for stealing his change. Eventually he was restrained until an emergency squad arrived; his blood glucose was found to be 30 mg/dL. He refused intravenous glucose treatment but took an oral glucose solution, after which he slowly began to improve. His family physician saw him in follow-up and learned that the patient had started using chromium picolinate 200 mcg two times a week and 300 mcg three times a week for bodybuilding. His episode of severe hypoglycemia was due to his use of chromium.[5]

Yeh et al. reviewed data from 108 clinical trials examining thirty-six herbs (single or in combination) and nine vitamin/mineral supplements involving 4,565 patients with impaired glucose tolerance or diabetes. The authors concluded that there was insufficient data to draw definitive conclusions regarding the efficacy of herbal supplements in controlling diabetes, but that the best evidence of efficacy for controlling blood glucose existed for *Coccinia indica* and American ginseng. Other supplements that showed promise were *Gymnema sylvestre*, aloe vera, vanadium, *Momordica charantia*, and nopal. Chromium was the most widely studied supplement for controlling blood glucose.[6]

Coccinia indica (ground ivy) is a creeping plant that grows wild in many parts of India and is used in traditional Indian Ayurvedic medicine for treating diabetes. Many formulations containing *Coccinia indica* are available in India and the United States. Cinnamon-6 herbal formulation (Herbal Pride) contains this herb as one of its many components. However, the Food and Drug Administration (FDA) has not evaluated the efficacy of this product in controlling type 2 diabetes.

Two long-term trials administering American ginseng for eight weeks reported decreases in fasting blood glucose. Glycosylated hemoglobin, another indicator of long-term glucose control, was also decreased in subjects taking American ginseng.[7] Various studies also indicate reduction in blood glucose after taking Korean or Asian ginseng.

The use of garlic in lowering blood sugar is controversial, although a few studies have shown positive effects. Fenugreek may also be effective in reducing blood sugars, but studies reported in the literature were not always well designed.[8]

Fig (*Ficus carica*) leaves may be effective in lowering blood sugar.[9] Chromium, a trace element, is required for the maintenance of normal metabolism of glucose. Chromium deficiency may cause glucose intolerance, although most diabetic patients are not chromium-deficient. Chromium picolinate may be effective in lowering blood glucose, although some studies showed no benefit. Herbal and dietary supplements that may reduce blood glucose are listed in Table 12.1.

TABLE 12.1: Herbal Remedies and Dietary Supplements That May Lower Blood Sugar

SUPPLEMENT	POSSIBLE EFFECTS
Aloe vera	Lowers sugar
Alpha-lipoic acid	May lower sugar
American ginseng	Lowers sugar
Asian ginseng	Lowers sugar, increases immune function
Bitter melon (*Momordica charantia*)	Lowers sugar
Chromium	Lowers sugar; increases insulin sensitivity
Coccinia indica (ground ivy)	Lowers sugar
Fenugreek seed	May lower sugar and lipids; may increase HDL ("good") cholesterol
Fig leaf	Lowers sugar
Garlic	Mixed results; may lower sugar and cholesterol
Gymnema sylvestre	Lowers sugar
Holy basil (*Ocimum sanctum*)	Lowers sugar
Korean ginseng	Lowers sugar
Manganese	Lowers sugar/no effect
Milk thistle	Lowers sugar
Nopal (*Opunita streptacantha*)	Lowers sugar
Prickly pear cactus	May lower sugar
Vanadium	Lowers sugar

Patients taking medications for controlling diabetes should not take any herbal supplement that may lower blood glucose without consulting their doctor. Many herbal supplements that lower glucose may act synergistically with these medications and lower glucose to critical levels, causing a medical emergency.

Kidney Function Tests

Kidney function, also called renal function, is usually determined by measuring concentrations of creatinine and urea in the blood. These concentrations, in relation to body-mass index, determine creatinine clearance, an indicator of healthy renal function. Many herbal remedies, especially Chinese weight-loss products, may cause acute renal failure, indicated by elevated creatinine and blood urea (measured as blood urea nitrogen or BUN). These supplements are discussed in detail in Chapter 7.

Blood Electrolytes Tests

Basically, our blood is composed of salt water (sodium chloride) and many other components such as potassium, calcium, and magnesium. Many trace elements such as copper, zinc, manganese, vanadium, chromium, cobalt, and selenium are essential for healthy living, while iron is an essential component of hemoglobin. Sodium chloride is the major electrolyte found in blood. A delicate balance of electrolytes in the blood is essential, and kidneys play an important role in maintaining that balance. Normal ranges of common electrolytes in serum are given in Table 12.2. If electrolyte balance in the blood is impaired, serious illness and even death can occur.

TABLE 12.2: Normal Serum Concentrations of Electrolytes

COMPONENT	NORMAL RANGE
Calcium	8.4–10.2 mg/dL
Chloride	98–106 mmol/L (millimoles per liter)
Magnesium	1.3–2.1 meq/L (milliequivalents per liter)
Potassium	3.5–5.1 mmol/L
Sodium	136–146 mmol/L

Several compounds found in herbs may cause electrolyte imbalance. Licorice is known to do so.

CASE STUDY

A seventy-seven-year-old man with a history of hypertension and high uric acid in the blood was admitted to the hospital. For ten years he had been taking a Chinese herbal supplement for allergy together with enalapril for controlling his blood pressure. Four months before this episode, he started taking another Chinese laxative for constipation. On admission, his serum electrolyte potassium was only 1.9 mmol/L (millimoles per liter), which was dangerously low. After discontinuation of both the Chinese remedies and therapy with potassium chloride, the patient recovered. The Chinese herb that the patient was taking contained glycyrrhizin, which is also the active component of licorice.[10]

Licorice is used in sweets and as a flavoring agent. The scientific literature indicates that single or occasional use of licorice-containing products may not cause any adverse effects. It is the chronic use of licorice-containing herbal supplements that may cause electrolyte imbalance.

> *Patients suffering from hypertension or taking spirolactone should not use licorice-containing herbal supplements.*

Thyroid Tests

Kelp, a type of seaweed, is rich in iodine. Our daily requirement of iodine is fulfilled because the salt we use has sufficient iodine added during its processing. Use of kelp supplement may cause iodine excess and result in thyroid problems, causing an abnormal thyroid profile. (See Chapter 7 for a more detailed discussion of kelp supplements.)

Therapeutic Drug Monitoring

Of the many drugs used today, only a small fraction (thirty to fifty) require routine monitoring, which means their blood concentrations need to be measured periodically in patients receiving them. These drugs have lower margins of safety. For example, only one or two tablets of Tylenol (acetaminophen) are needed for headache relief. In order for severe liver failure—which is an adverse effect of acetaminophen—to occur, you would have to take fifteen to twenty tablets at once. On the other hand, digoxin, used to treat various heart conditions, can be toxic if used regularly at normally prescribed dosages. Therefore, your doctor would routinely monitor your blood digoxin levels in order to prevent digoxin toxicity.

Therapeutic drug monitorings are important laboratory tests, and herbals may affect some of these tests, such as the monitoring of digoxin. In addition, these laboratory tests can also help physicians identify any unwanted interaction between an herb and a drug. Table 12.3 lists common drugs that may require therapeutic drug monitoring.

TABLE 12.3: Common Drugs That Require Routine Therapeutic Drug Monitoring

CLASS OF MEDICATION	DRUG	TRADE NAME
Anticonvulsants	Phenytoin	Dilantin
	Carbamazepine	Tegretol
	Phenobarbital	Solfoton
	Primidone	Mysoline
	Valproic acid	Depakote
Antiasthmatics	Theophylline	Elixophyllin, Theo-24
Antidepressants	Amitriptyline	Elavil
	Doxepin	Sinequan
	Imipramine	Tofranil
	Clomipramine	Anafranil
	Lithium	Lithane
Antineoplastics (chemo-therapy drugs)	Methotrexate†	Amethopterin, Mexate, Rheumatrex
Cardioactive drugs	Digoxin	Lanoxin
	Procainamide	Procan
	Quinidine sulfate	Quinaglute
	Quinidine gluconate	Quinidex
	Lidocaine hydrochloride	Xylocaine
Immunosuppressants	Cyclosporine	Sandimmune
	Tacrolimus	Prograf
	Mycophenolic acid	CellCept

† May not require monitoring if used in low dosage for the treatment of rheumatoid arthritis.

The above listed drugs are the common drugs that are monitored in most hospitals. Physicians in specialized clinics may monitor other drugs; for example, selected antiretrovirals in HIV clinics.

St. John's wort, an herbal antidepressant, induces liver enzymes that metabolize many drugs and thus reduces serum concentrations, causing treatment failure.

In one report by Ahmed et al., three heart-transplant recipients who previously had desirable blood concentrations of cyclosporine (100–150 ng/mL) showed significantly lower levels of cyclosporine in their blood tests (performed every six to eight weeks) after starting to take St. John's wort. They denied skipping any dose of cyclosporine, having episodes of vomiting or diarrhea, or taking any new medication except for St. John's wort. Two patients were taking one tablet (usually 300 mg of dry extract) each of St. John's wort every day, and their cyclosporine levels fell to 64 ng/mL (nanograms per milliliter) and 63 ng/mL, respectively. The third patient, who was taking two tablets of St. John's wort each day, showed a very low cyclosporine level of 35 ng/mL in their blood.[11] Although none of the patients experienced organ rejection, acute organ rejection in patients taking St. John's wort has been reported. This is due to reduced levels of the anti-rejection drug cyclosporine. St. John's wort increases the metabolism of cyclosporine and may cause treatment failure. Many other drugs also interact with St. John's wort. (Please see Chapter 7 for more details.)

CASE STUDY

Digoxin Monitoring

Herbal supplements may falsely increase or decrease the serum digoxin concentration measured by an immunoassay test due to interference with the assay antibody (a bioactive chemical used in the test).

A seventy-four-year-old man undergoing digoxin therapy had maintained therapeutic levels between 0.9 to 2.2 ng/mL over a period of ten years. However, after ingestion of Siberian ginseng, his serum digoxin level increased to 5.2 ng/mL, but there were no signs or symptoms of digoxin toxicity. After he stopped taking the ginseng, his serum digoxin level returned to previous therapeutic levels. The patient resumed taking ginseng, and several months later his serum digoxin level was again elevated. Digoxin therapy was maintained at a constant daily dose, the ginseng was stopped once again, and the serum digoxin concentration returned to a therapeutic level.[12]

CASE STUDY

Interference of herbal supplements with digoxin immunoassay may be high or moderate. The traditional Chinese medicines Chan Su and Liu Shen Wan, and oleander-containing herbal supplements cause very significant interference in serum digoxin measurement by immunoassays. On the other hand, Asian ginseng, danshen, and the Indian Ayurvedic medicine ashwagandha cause only moderate interference that may not significantly alter digoxin values.[13] Table 12.4 lists herbal supplements that may interfere with serum digoxin assay.

TABLE 12.4: Interference of Herbal Products in Therapeutic Digoxin Monitoring

HERBAL PRODUCT	MAGNITUDE OF INTERFERENCE
American ginseng	Moderate to low
Ashwagandha	Moderate to low
Asian ginseng	Moderate to low
Chan Su	High
Liu Shen Wan	High to moderate
Oleander-containing herbs	High
Siberian ginseng	Mixed results

Patients Using Herbal Remedies During Surgery

The use of herbal remedies by patients undergoing elective surgery is a significant problem due to potential interactions between herbal supplements and anesthetic, as well as a risk of bleeding during and after surgery.[14] Multiple authors have made suggestions regarding the cessation of use of herbal supplements prior to surgery. Ang-Lee et al. recommend that garlic and ginseng be discontinued at least seven days prior to surgery because both herbs have been reported to cause bleeding. Ginkgo biloba should also be discontinued three days prior to surgery because it inhibits platelet aggregation, causing bleeding. Kava should be discontinued at least twenty-four hours before surgery because it can increase the sedative effect of anesthetics. Ma Huang (ephedra) should also be discontinued twenty-four hours prior to surgery because it increases blood pressure and heart rate. St. John's wort should be discontinued five days prior to surgery because it induces liver enzymes that metabolize drugs and may significantly reduce their concentrations. This is particularly important for transplant surgery because cyclosporine is used as an immunosuppressant.[15] The American Society of Anesthesiologists recommends that all herbal supplements be discontinued two to three weeks before elective surgery.[16]

Herbal Remedies Contaminated with Western Drugs

Many herbal remedies originating in Asian countries are contaminated with Western drugs or heavy metals. Therefore, the unexpected presence of a drug or a high concentration of a particular heavy metal may be encountered in laboratory test results for a patient taking such supplements. This is a serious problem with imported traditional Chinese herbal products and Ayurvedic medicines originating from India. Chapter 13 is dedicated to these critical issues.

Conclusion

Many herbal supplements may distort the results of common, standard medical tests and may confuse your clinician.[17] You need to know which herbal remedies may affect your lab tests so you can exercise proper caution before you go in for a routine medical checkup.

It is vital that you disclose your use of herbal supplements to your doctor, because if you do so, your doctor can effectively interpret any unexpected laboratory results and advise you about whether you should discontinue use of that herbal product.

Herbal Remedies That Are Misidentified or Contaminated with Heavy Metals or Western Drugs

T oxicity from a relatively safe herbal supplement may occur because another, cheaper herbal supplement was used in its place. Some traditional Chinese medicines imported from Asian countries and Ayurvedic medicines imported from India may be contaminated with heavy metals. Problems with Indian Ayurvedic medicines are discussed in detail in Chapter 14.

Misidentification of Herbal Supplement

Misidentification of an herbal supplement may produce serious adverse effects. Good communication between regulators, manufacturers, and practitioners is important to avoid toxic effects of herbal remedies.[1]

Usually, dried herbs and roots are cheaper than processed liquid extracts or capsules, and many people buy unprocessed herbs in order to save money. Unfortunately, chopped herbs are more difficult to identify, and misidentification may occur.[2] Moreover, the concentration of active ingredients in unprocessed herbs may vary from one season to another, resulting in a lower- or higher-than-intended dosage. When a reputable manufacturer prepares herbal supplements, care is exercised to properly identify the herb. In addition, standardization of the active ingredient in that herbal supplement is used as a quality-control measure. For example, most commercial preparations of St. John's wort are usually standardized to 0.3 percent hypericin, an active ingredient.

Many cases of herb misidentification have been reported. Plantain is an edible fruit, and its young leaves have long been used in folk medicine for treating cold and cough, lowering cholesterol, and other purposes. Plantain is a safe herbal product, but in 1998 two case reports were published describing serious toxicity due to use of plantain products. Both patients showed significant amounts of the heart medication digoxin in their blood, although neither of the patients was taking digoxin. Both patients experienced serious cardiac toxicity that required hospitalization. Later, it was found that six hundred pounds of plantain imported from Germany into the United States was contaminated with cardiac glycosides because these products contained *Digitalis lantana*, a species of foxglove. Digoxin is one of the components of this plant, and digoxin, along with other cardiac glycosides, caused serious intoxication in these two patients.[3] In 2006 our laboratory analyzed several batches of commercially available plantain and found no contamination of cardiac glycoside.[4]

> *If you want to take an herbal supplement, it is better to buy a liquid product or capsule from a reputable manufacturer than to consume the herb in its raw state.*

The use of ginseng does not cause unusual hair growth (androgenization). Yet maternal ingestion of Siberian ginseng once caused androgenization in a newborn, who was born with thick, black hair over its entire forehead and pubic area and showed swollen, red nipples. It was discovered that the Siberian ginseng was contaminated with Chinese silk vine, which is toxic to the liver.[5]

CASE STUDY

A nineteen-year-old farm laborer presented to the hospital with a twenty-four-hour history of abdominal discomfort and vomiting, dizziness, blurred vision, and malaise. He had mistakenly ingested seven leaves of foxglove, thinking it was comfrey, because foxglove leaf and comfrey leaf have a similar appearance. He was not exposed to digoxin as far as he knew, but his serum digoxin level was 3.7 ng/mL (nanogram per milliliter). This was consistent with foxglove poisoning, and such a high digoxin level in the blood could be fatal. Fortunately, he recovered following supportive treatment.[6]

This case report indicates the danger of self-identification of herbal plants for consumption.

In 1993, rapidly progressing kidney damage was reported in a group of young women who were taking pills containing Chinese herbs while attending a weight-loss clinic in Belgium. It was discovered that one prescription Chinese herb had been replaced with another Chinese herb containing aristolochic acid, a known kidney toxin. (Please see Chapter 7 for more discussion.)

Misidentification of Wild Mushrooms

Although not related to this topic, self-identification of wild mushrooms for consumption as a food is dangerous. Many Amanita genuses of mushrooms are very poisonous and may cause fatal liver failure or severe liver failure requiring liver transplant. Madhok et al. reported three cases of severe liver toxicity due to ingestion of wild mushroom. Fortunately, none of the subjects died.[7] Mushroom poisoning often occurs even to experienced collectors. The increasing popularity of natural foods has led to an increased incidence of wild-mushroom poisonings among the general population. In one case report, a grandmother with more than thirty years of self-taught expertise in identifying wild mushrooms prepared a mushroom dish for herself and three family members. A three-year-old child died from mushroom poisoning, but the others recovered.[8]

Unintentional Versus Intentional Contamination of Herbal Products

Contamination of herbal supplements with heavy metals, pesticides, or Western drugs may be intentional or unintentional. For example, a group of investigators detected colchicine (a toxic natural product used in treating gout) in the placental blood samples of five out of twenty-four women. All five of these women were taking herbal supplements, most notably ginkgo biloba and echinacea, during pregnancy but never took any colchicine-containing medication. The other nineteen women who had no colchicine in the placental blood did not take any herbal supplement. The investigators analyzed several brands of ginkgo and echinacea obtained from local herbal stores and found measurable amounts of colchicine in those products. This was probably an accidental contamination because it was unlikely that a manufacturer would have contaminated a product with colchicine, a toxic substance.[9] Usually, colchicine is not found in these herbal supplements. The contamination of plantain with foxglove (*Digitalis lantana*), described earlier, also appeared to be unintentional, as our laboratory was unable to detect any digitalis in several plantain preparations we analyzed later.

Similarly, the presence of heavy metals in many traditional Chinese medicines may be related to growing those herbs in contaminated soil or problems with the manufacturing process, but it appears to be unintentional. The same is true for Indian Ayurvedic medicines. In addition, many Ayurvedic medicines contain heavy metals as active ingredients. Nevertheless, if heavy-metal contamination of such supplements is significant, toxicity may result from their consumption. Contamination of herbal supplements with pesticides is another example of unintentional contamination.

On the other hand, certain adulterations of herbal products are certainly intentional. Deliberate contamination takes place when the necessary natural ingredients are expensive or in short supply or when a manufacturer wants to intensify a particular pharmacological effect by adulterating the supplement with a Western drug. The use of pharmaceutical-grade caffeine to supplement kola nuts is an example of intentional adulteration of an herbal supplement and is a violation of the 1994 U.S. Dietary Supplement Health and Education Act.

Heavy-Metal Contamination of Herbal Supplements

Contamination of herbal supplements with heavy metals, especially herbal products imported into the United States, is a very serious problem. Lead, mercury, arsenic, and cadmium poisoning following consumption of herbal supplements or herbal vitamins manufactured in various Asian, South American, and African countries has been documented. Based on a current literature review, it appears that many contaminated products reported are Indian Ayurvedic medicines and traditional Asian medicines, including Chinese medicines. In a recent report, Saper et al. concluded that one-fifth of Ayurvedic medicines manufactured in both the United States and India (purchased via the Internet) contained detectable lead, mercury, or arsenic.[10] The presence of heavy metals in Ayurvedic medicines produced in the United States may be due to the fact that heavy metals are a part of the active components in the formula. In another report, the authors analyzed many herbal products used in Brazil and observed the presence of cadmium, mercury, and lead.[11] Cooper et al. reported that of 247 traditional Chinese medicines, 5–15 percent were contaminated with arsenic, 5 percent with lead, and 65 percent with mercury. Some preparations even exceeded the tolerable daily intake for males and females for arsenic (four products for males, five products for female), lead (one product for males and two for females), and mercury (five products for males and seven products for females). These products exceeded limits by as much as 2,760-fold, thus posing substantial risk of poisoning.[12] However, it is also obvious from this report that only a small fraction of traditional Chinese medicines are contaminated with high amounts of heavy metals that pose serious health risks.

> *How can a consumer differentiate contaminated products from noncon-*
> *taminated ones? Sadly, only chemical analysis in a sophisticated laboratory*
> *can identify contaminated products.*

The most confusing aspect of heavy-metal contamination of imported herbal supplements is trying to obtain an estimate of what percentage of such supplements is contaminated. Obi et al. reported that 100 percent of all Nigerian herbal supplements studied were contaminated with heavy metals including cadmium, copper, iron, nickel, selenium, zinc, lead, and mercury. The authors warned of the potential of heavy-metal toxicity from use of such herbal supplements.[13] Another report analyzed traditional herbal remedies purchased in the United States, Vietnam, and China. It was observed that the Asian remedies evaluated contained arsenic, lead, and mercury that ranged from toxic (49 percent of the products) to those exceeding public-health guidelines of maximum tolerable limits (74 percent of the products). This implies that the majority of Asian remedies analyzed by these investigators were contaminated with heavy metals.[14]

Heavy-Metal Toxicity

Lead poisoning is the most commonly reported heavy-metal poisoning following consumption of traditional Asian medicines. Lead has no known physiological role in the human body, but it has a unique ability to mimic other physiologically important metal ions such as iron, zinc, and calcium. Because of this ability, lead can bind to important enzymes and proteins and thus disrupt their normal biological functions. Lead interferes with the biosynthesis of heme (the nonprotein part of hemoglobin that contains iron), which is essential for the production of hemoglobin, thus causing moderate to severe anemia depending on how much lead is in the blood. Lead poisoning sometimes mimics the symptoms and biochemical tests of another disease known as porphyria. Lead is removed from the body extremely slowly and tends to deposit in bones. Symptoms of lead poisoning include abdominal pain, nausea, vomiting, lethargy, metallic taste in the mouth, weight loss, and neurological problems. Chronic lead poisoning in children is more dangerous than in adults because lead interferes with normal development and may cause decreased IQ.

Lead poisoning is treated by appropriate chelation therapy, and it is also important to identify the source of lead exposure and remove that source from the patient's environment. In a case of lead toxicity due to ingestion of traditional Asian medicines, discontinuation of the medication is essential in order to eliminate the source of lead exposure.

Arsenic poisons people by inhibiting the essential enzymes responsible for metabolism. Symptoms include violent stomach pain, excessive saliva production, hoarseness, and difficulty in speech. Severe or chronic poisoning leads to delirium and, if untreated, may also be fatal. However, there are excellent chelating agents for treating arsenic poisoning.

One source of arsenic poisoning is drinking-well water if the groundwater is contaminated with arsenic. The largest reported mass poisoning by arsenic from drinking water occurred in Bangladesh. In the 1970s and 1980s international development organizations, including UNICEF, sponsored the installation of more than ten million wells in Bangladesh so that villagers did not need to drink water from rivers, ponds, or any other surface water source. Unfortunately, soils were not tested and it was later discovered that the well water was contaminated with arsenic; in some specimens the arsenic level in the water was five or ten times the safe limit recommended by the World Health Organization. In a 1999 survey it was found that 27 million people had been exposed to high levels of arsenic over many years, while another 50 million had been exposed to moderate amounts. The symptoms of chronic exposure to arsenic start with blackening of the hands and feet, a condition that later spreads over the body, causing sores and even gangrene. Eventually, arsenic poisoning causes cardiovascular and reproductive damage as well as bladder, lung, and other types of cancer. Arsenic exposure in children causes learning disabilities.[15] Arsenic poisoning as a result of drinking contaminated water has also been reported in India, China, Taiwan, Chile, Thailand, and Argentina.[16]

Mercury poisoning may occur as a result of exposure to elemental mercury, inorganic mercury, or organic mercury. Other than contaminated Asian medicines, another major source of mercury exposure is contaminated fish. Among the common symptoms of mercury poisoning are peripheral neuropathy (severe itching, burning, or pain in hands and feet), skin discoloration (pink cheeks, fingernails, and toes), and swelling. Mercury poisoning requires quick medical attention.

CASE STUDY   A fifty-four-year-old woman was referred to the University of California, Davis, Occupational Medicine Clinic with a two-year history of alopecia and memory loss. She also complained of rash, fatigue, nausea, and vomiting that made her unable to work full-time. She admitted taking a daily kelp supplement. Her urine sample showed high amounts of arsenic, and when her kelp supplement was analyzed, arsenic was detected in it as well. After she stopped taking the kelp supplement, her symptoms resolved and eventually her blood and urine tests showed no arsenic. In order to determine the extent of arsenic contamination in kelp supplements, the investigators analyzed nine supplements from the local market and detected arsenic in eight of the nine samples.[17]

CASE STUDY   A forty-five-year-old Korean man developed abdominal colic, muscle pain, and fatigue and was hospitalized. His blood lead level was elevated to 76 mcg/100 mL (normal level: less than 10 mcg/100 mL of blood). No occupational source of lead was detected. The patient had been taking the Chinese herbal preparation Hai Ge Fen (clamshell powder) for four weeks prior to admission. Analysis of the clamshell powder showed the presence of lead, and it was concluded that the lead poisoning in this patient was due to ingestion of the Chinese medicine.[18]

Heavy-metal contamination of traditional Chinese and other Asian medicines may be related to the formulation of a proprietary product, manufacturing practices, or the accumulation of heavy metals in plants due to contaminated soil. Barthwal et al. demonstrated that levels of heavy metal differed in the same medicinal plant collected from environmentally different sites of the same city. The authors concluded that medicinal plants should be tested for contamination before processing.[19]

Pesticide Contamination of Herbal Supplements

Contamination of vegetables and food products with pesticides is a common problem worldwide. Herbal supplements are not free from such contamination. Today the use of pesticides is inevitable in the cultivation of herbal plants in many countries due to the growing demands for herbal products worldwide.

There are several reports in the literature of contamination of traditional Chinese medicines with pesticides. In one study, the authors analyzed 280 specimens of 30 traditional Chinese medicines and observed that pesticide contamination was widespread. However, concentrations of pesticides exceeded tolerable limits in only four samples.[20] Even the banned pesticide DDT has been detected in Chinese medicine,[21] although pesticide poisoning from the ingestion of Chinese medicine has been reported very infrequently.

CASE STUDY

A sixty-eight-year-old man presented at the hospital with the classic symptoms of pesticide poisoning (cholinergic syndrome), in which the acetylcholinesterase activity in his blood cells was reduced to 50 percent of normal value. The patient was taking *Flemingia macrophylla* and ginseng. He recovered after treatment with the antidote atropine. It was believed that pesticide poisoning was due to ingestion of a contaminated herb.[22]

Herbal Supplements Contaminated with Western Drugs

Certain proprietary Chinese medicines manufactured in various Asian countries may be contaminated with undisclosed Western drugs, even banned drugs. The addition of pharmaceuticals to Chinese herbal products is a serious problem. In one report, the authors analyzed 2,069 samples of traditional Chinese medicines collected from eight hospitals in Taiwan. In 618 samples (23.7 percent), they encountered undeclared Western pharmaceuticals, most commonly caffeine, acetaminophen, indomethacin, hydrochlorothiazide, and prednisolone.[23] Most of these supplements were used to alleviate pain, inflammation, or symptoms of arthritis. Pharmaceuticals such as acetaminophen, indomethacin, and prednisolone can achieve those therapeutic effects. In addition, use of a steroid such as prednisolone is dangerous without medical advice. Because contamination by these Western drugs is not disclosed in these herbal supplements, serious toxicity may result due to drug overdose. Adulteration of these traditional Chinese medicines is certainly intentional and violates American laws. Unfortunately, some of these products eventually come to the U.S. market.

CASE STUDY

Lau et al. reported a case of phenytoin poisoning in a patient following use of Chinese medicines. This patient was treated with valproic acid, carbamazepine, and phenobarbital for epilepsy but was never prescribed phenytoin. She consumed three bottles of a Chinese proprietary medicine in addition to her prescribed medicines. She showed a toxic phenytoin level of 48.5 mcg/mL in her blood, which was potentially life-threatening. Analysis of her Chinese medicines showed adulteration with phenytoin, although the product leaflet stated that the preparation contained only Chinese herbs.[24]

CASE STUDY

A twenty-year-old athlete tested positive for benzodiazepines (a group of drugs used in treating anxiety, depression, or sleeplessness) on a random drug screening, and later the presence of diazepam, a benzodiazepine, in her urine specimen was confirmed. The student denied use of any illicit drug or prescription medication containing benzodiazepines. However, she admitted that she was taking a Chinese herbal product obtained from her hometown chiropractor in Ohio. She supplied that Chinese "miracle herb" for analysis. The presence of diazepam, a prescription medicine, was confirmed. The chiropractor had obtained the product from a supplier located in Hutchinson, Kansas, but was unaware that it was contaminated with the Western drug.[25]

CASE STUDY

A twenty-five-year-old woman came to the emergency room with severe abdominal pain of two weeks' duration and a one-day history of nausea and vomiting. She had been taking high-dose ibuprofen, which she had discontinued five days earlier. She had also been taking a Brazilian weight-loss supplement, Emagrece Sim, which she purchased over the Internet and had discontinued two weeks earlier. Her friends, who were taking the same supplement, felt similar symptoms. Her urine tested positive for amphetamine, a narcotic. She denied abuse of amphetamine, and it was suspected that the expensive diet pills ($270 for one month's supply) might be contaminated with amphetamine. The bright yellow-and-orange diet capsules were brought to the hospital by her friends, and upon analysis, the presence of a banned amphetamine derivative (5-cyanoethyl-amphetamine) was confirmed.[26]

CASE STUDY

A fifty-six-year-old Indonesian tourist came to a hospital in Perth, Australia, with severely low blood glucose: 37.9 mg/100 mL (normal is 70–99 mg/dL). He was unable to speak, but his wife informed the doctor that he had arrived from Jakarta three days earlier and was suffering flulike symptoms. He was treated immediately with a glucagon injection. Later he was alert and his blood glucose level was stabilized to 77.4 mg/dL. But his blood glucose dropped again, and an infusion of glucose was initiated. Eventually, it was found that the patient spoke fluent English and that he had non-insulin-dependent diabetes, which he controlled by diet. He was not taking any diabetes medication but had been taking a traditional herbal product, Zhen Qi, which he purchased in Malaysia, for five years. The label on the bottle listed ginseng, pearl, ram's horn, bark, and frog extract as active ingredients. However, analysis of the supplement demonstrated the presence of the Western diabetic medication glibenclamide. His severely low glucose was probably due to the contamination of the herbal supplement with this Western drug.[27]

CASE STUDY

A forty-two-year-old woman developed severe liver failure after having ingested an unknown quantity of an herbal product over a period of four months. Unfortunately, she died forty-eight hours later. Analysis of the herbal supplement showed the presence of fenfluramine, N-nitroso-fenfluramine, nicotinamide, and thyroid extract. Fenfluramine is a banned drug in the United States but has no known toxic effect to the liver. However, N-nitroso-fenfluramine has known liver toxicity, and it was speculated that that might be the cause of her liver failure.[28]

These case reports clearly establish the danger of using traditional Chinese herbal supplements, which may be contaminated with Western drugs. Ku et al., using a sophisticated analytic method called high-performance capillary electrophoresis, observed four antidiabetic medications (acetohexamide, chlorpropamide, glibenclamide, and tolbutamide) present as adulterants in various traditional Chinese medicines.[29] Even drugs that are banned by the FDA are found in some traditional Chinese medicines. Another study by Ku et al. reported the presence of the banned drugs phenylpropanolamine and fenfluramine, along with methamphetamine, as adulterants in some traditional Chinese medicines. Other drugs such as clobenzorex, diethylpropion, and phentermine were found as well.[30]

CASE STUDY

A twelve-year-old boy developed aplastic anemia (a potentially fatal illness in which bone marrow cannot produce enough blood cells to replenish blood) due to intake of an herbal supplement containing the banned drug phenylbutazone. Phenylbutazone was not listed as an ingredient, and no warning was provided on the supplement's label.[31]

Common Western drugs found in traditional Asian medicines are listed in Table 13.1.

TABLE 13.1: Undeclared Western Drugs Encountered in Traditional Asian Medicines

CLASS OF MEDICATION	DRUG
Analgesics (nonsteroidal anti-inflammatories)	Diclofenac, ibuprofen, indomethacin, mefenamic acid, methyl salicylate
Anticonvulsants	Carbamazepine, phenytoin, valproic acid
Antidiabetics	Acetohexamide, chlorpropamide, glibenclamide, tolbutamide
Banned agents	5-cyanoethyl-amphetamine, fenfluramine, phenylbutazone, phenylpropanolamine
Benzodiazepines	Diazepam
Diuretics	Hydrochlorothiazide
Erectile-dysfunction drugs	Sildenafil (Viagra)
Muscle relaxants	Chlorzoxazone
Pain medications	Acetaminophen, phenacetin
Steroids	Clobetasol, dexamethasone, fluocinolone , prednisolone
Stimulants	Caffeine, phenacetin

Although most reports of Western drug contamination refer to traditional Chinese medicine, many weight-loss products manufactured in the United States may also be contaminated with Western drugs, including drugs that are banned by the FDA. In November 1999 the FDA warned the public regarding the use of Triax Metabolic Accelerator, a weight-loss product manufactured by Syntrax Innovations, because it contained triiodoacetic acid, which may cause heart attack or stroke. In 2004 the FDA warned people about using Liqiang 4, which is manufactured in China but distributed by Bugle International of California, because the product contained glyburide, a medication used by diabetic patients to lower blood glucose. In January 2009 the FDA determined that many dietary supplements marketed for weight loss are contaminated with various drugs such as sibutramine, rimonabant, phenytoin, phenolphthalein, and bumetanide. Sibutramine is a Schedule 4 drug (meaning it has potential for abuse or dependence) that is approved to treat obesity. Rimonabant is not approved by the FDA. Phenolphthalein was used in over-the-counter laxatives, but in 1999 the FDA determined that it is not safe for human consumption. Bumetanide is used in prescription diuretics. Phenytoin is a prescription anticonvulsant. Legally, no manufacturer can add a Western drug to a dietary supplement. A list of these contaminated products is presented in Table 13.2.

TABLE 13.2: Weight-Loss Products Contaminated with Various Drugs

WEIGHT-LOSS PRODUCT	DRUG FOUND
2 Day Diet, 2 Day Diet Slim Advance, 2x Powerful Slimming, 3 Day Diet, 3 Days Fit, 3x Slimming Power, 5x Imelda Perfect Slimming, 7 Day Herbal Slim, 7 Days Diet, 7 Diet, 7 Diet Day/Night Formula, 21 Double Slim, 24 Hours Diet, 999 Fitness Essence, Body Creator, Body Shaping, Body Slimming, Cosmo Slim, Extrim Plus, Extrim Plus 24 Hour Reburn, Fasting Diet, GMP, Imelda Fat Reducer, JM Fat Reducer, Lida DaiDaihua, Meili, Meizitang, Miaozi, MeiMiaoQianZiJianNang, Maiozi Slim Capsules, Natural Model, Perfect Slim, Perfect Slim Up, Powerful Slim, ProSlim Plus, Reduce Weight, Sana Plus, Slim 3 in 1, Slim 3 in 1 Extra Slim Formula, Slim 3 in 1 Extra Slim Waist Formula, Slim 3 in 1 M18 Royal Diet, Slim 3 in 1 Slim Formula, Slim Burn, Slim Express 4 in 1, Slim Express 360, Slim Fast,* Slim Tech, Slim Up, Slim Waist Formula, Slim Waistline, Slimbionic, Sliminate, Slimming Formula, Somotrim, Super Fat Burner, Super Slimming, Trim 2 Plus, Triple Slim, Venom Hyperdrive 3.0, Waist Strength Formula, Xsvelten	Sibutramine
Phyto Shape	Rimonabant
3 x Slimming Power, Extrim Plus	Sibutramine, phenytoin
8 Factors Diet, Fatloss Slimming, Imelda Perfect Slim, Perfect Slim 5x, Royal Slimming Formula, Superslim, Zhen De Shou	Sibubtramin and phenolphthalein
Starcaps	Bumetanide

* This product should not be confused with the line of meal-replacement and related products marketed as conventional foods under the brand name Slim-Fast. The manufacturer of Slim-Fast, Unilever United States, maintains that the Slim Fast product that appears on this list is not in any way associated with, sponsored or approved by, or otherwise related in any way to the Slim-Fast brand of meal-replacement and related products. (Source: http://www.fda.gov./Drugs/ResourcesforYou/Consumers/QuestionAnswers/ucm136187.htm, accessed 6/1/2009).

Traditional Chinese Medicine: Is There Any Good News?

Traditional Chinese medicine has been practiced for more than three thousand years in China, and today, both Western and traditional Chinese medicine are practiced side by side in many hospital facilities. In traditional Chinese medicine, typically more than one herb is prescribed by an experienced herbalist so that the side effects of one herb can be neutralized by another. However, in the United States many people take one Chinese herb based on a conversation with friends and may experience toxicity. If you wish to take any Chinese herbal supplement, the first step is to talk to a qualified Chinese herbalist or a Doctor of Oriental Medicine.

Although a fraction of traditional Chinese medicines originating in Asian countries are contaminated with heavy metals or Western drugs, a significant portion of traditional Asian medicines reaching the United States market is free from adulteration. Unfortunately, there is no simple way to distinguish an adulterated product from an unadulterated one. One choice is to see if any American or European manufacturer offers the product. Otherwise, talking to an experienced Chinese herbalist may inform you about which manufacturers in Asian countries are more reputable and which products are more likely to be free from contamination.

There is a wealth of knowledge in traditional Chinese medicine and many reports in the literature establishing therapeutic benefits of traditional Chinese herbs in treating challenging diseases such as cancer and AIDS. For example, cyclotides isolated from the Chinese medicinal herb *Viola yedoensis* showed promising results as an anti-HIV agent.[32] A detailed discussion of traditional Chinese medicines is beyond the scope of this book, but there are many excellent books available on the subject.

The good news about traditional Chinese medicine is that the government of China is actively funding research projects with the goal of discovering new therapies based on the wealth of knowledge in traditional Chinese medicine. In 1956, Shanghai University of Traditional Chinese Medicine was founded. It has since grown significantly, becoming a reputed international research center. The China Academy of Chinese Medical Sciences is another very reputable institute devoted to rediscovering gems in traditional Chinese medicines. U.S. scientists are also taking an interest in traditional Chinese medicine. In June 2006 top health officials in the United States and China signed a memorandum of understanding to collaborate on research in integrative traditional Chinese medicine. Basic and clinical research on herbal supplements and acupuncture will be pursued by the investigators in this joint venture. This memorandum was signed by Dr. Stephen E. Straus, director of the National Center for Complementary and Alternative Medicine (National Institutes of Health), Sun Hong, deputy director general of the Ministry of Science and Technology, People's Republic of China, and other top officials (http://nccam.nih.gov/research/oihr/intent.htm). As purified products are isolated and developed as new drugs, horizons will open up in treating disease based on traditional knowledge. Moreover, these new drugs will be manufactured following rigorous standards and will be free from any contamination. As more and more papers are published on the adulteration of traditional Asian medicines, government agencies in these countries will increase vigilance. By imposing strict penalties they can deter certain corrupt manufacturers from adulterating traditional Chinese herbs with Western drugs.

It is worth noting that an increasing number of Western pharmaceuticals (and possibly herbal supplements) are being manufactured *in* China. Some reports estimate that up to 20 percent of finished drugs and more than 40 percent of the active ingredients of pills made in the United States come from India and China, and these numbers could double in the next twenty years.

Conclusion

Adulteration of traditional Asian medicines, Indian Ayurvedic medicines, and folk medicines originating in Africa and South American countries with various heavy metals and pesticides is in most instances unintentional. Nevertheless, if amounts of heavy-metal or pesticide contaminations are substantial in certain preparations, toxicity requiring medical attention may result. On the other hand, adulteration of certain traditional Chinese medicines with Western drugs is clearly intentional on the part of some manufacturers, and these practices are in violation of the 1994 Dietary Supplement Health and Education Act of the United States. Herbal supplements manufactured by reputable U.S. herbal companies are mostly free from such contamination. In addition, American manufacturers adopt more quality-control procedures in producing herbal supplements, and to the knowledge of this author, there is no report of intentional adulteration of any herbal supplement with pharmaceutical-grade drugs by any American manufacturer. There are many excellent references on this subject in the medical literature.[33]

CHAPTER 14

An Introduction to Ayurvedic Medicine

Ayurveda, "the science of life," is a traditional Indian system of medicine that probably originated in around 1900 B.C.[1] The earliest text of Ayurveda was probably written several centuries before the birth of Christ. The two most famous texts are the *Sushruta Samhita* and the *Charaka Samhita*. Today, Ayurvedic medicine is practiced in India along with Western medicine. Ayurvedic medicine is taught in more than 150 Ayurvedic medical colleges in India, and the curriculums are approved by appropriate accreditation agencies. Some of these Ayurvedic medical colleges are government institutions, for example, the Ayurvedic Medical College at Mysore. In India, training in Ayurvedic medicine may take up to five years, and after successful completion an individual is awarded a BAMS (Bachelor of Ayurvedic Medicine and Surgery) degree. Postgraduate education in Ayurveda is also available in India from more than thirty institutions (http://nccam.nih.gov/health/ayurveda). The Medical Council of India, a federal agency, actively supports research in Ayurvedic medicine. In the United States, Ayurvedic medicine is considered a form of complementary and alternative medicine (CAM).

The Basic Principles of Ayurvedic Medicine

Ayurveda is probably the most ancient form of personalized medicine in which treating the patient is as important as treating the disease. It is based on the belief that humans, as a part of the natural world, should live in harmony with the universe. The human body is seen as composed of the five elements of the cosmos: fire, water, air, earth, and space. (These elements are metaphorical.) For example, fire represents the force in nature that produces heat and radiates light; water is the force of life that holds things together; air and earth/space represent the spatial and physical environment.[2] The key concept is that when the mind and body are in harmony with the universe, the interaction is natural and wholesome. Disease occurs when this harmony is disrupted; the disruption may be physical, emotional, or spiritual in nature, or it may be from a combination of these.

The constitution of the body is called *prakriti*, and this is an inherent characteristic of an individual. Three life forces, or *doshas*, determine a person's chance of becoming sick; sickness occurs when the *doshas* are out of balance. The three *doshas* are *vata*, *pitta*, and *kapha*. The *vata* represents air, *pitta* represents elements of fire and water, and *kapha* combines the elements of water and earth. *Pitta* can also be translated to mean "bile." The body contains seven elements, known as *dhatus*. These *dhatus* are summarized in Table 14.1. In addition to *vata*, *pitta*, and *kapha*, which control the body, three *gunas* (qualities) control the mind. These *gunas* are *sattva*, *rajas*, and *tamas*. People with *sattva guna* are more spiritual in nature than people with *rajas* or *tamas*. The energy metabolism is called *agni*, and the three excretory products are feces, urine, and sweat. Because *prakriti* differs from one person to another, Ayurvedic treatment, both in its course and duration, is tailored to the individual.

TABLE 14.1: The Seven Elements (*Dhatus*) of the Body

DHATU	WHAT IT MEANS
Asthi	Bones
Majja	Bone marrow and nervous system
Mamsa	Muscles and tissue
Med	Fatty tissue
Rakta	Blood
Rasa	Plasma and skin
Shukra	Reproductive system

Diagnosis in Ayurvedic medicine is from a holistic perspective and involves a thorough questioning of the individual to obtain a family history and also a physical examination of the patient. Physical examination includes listening to the heart, the lungs, and the intestine, feeling the skin and key parts of the body, and examining pulse and the tongue. Based on the diagnosis, a course of treatment is prescribed that may include a special diet, change of lifestyle, exercise, massage, prayer, and appropriate herbal supplements.

There are four main categories of disease treatment in Ayurveda: cleansing (*shodan*), palliation (*shaman*), rejuvenation (*rasayana*), and mental health (*satvajaya*). Cleansing or detoxification of the body, called *panchakarma*, is an important part of Ayurvedic treatment (see Table 14.2) and includes vomiting, purging, enema, administration of herbs through the nasal passage, and bleeding.[3] However, due to the medical risk involved, bleeding is not performed in the modern practice of *panchakarma*. Palliation treatment can be performed in a variety of ways, including using herbs such as ginger, cinnamon, and black pepper, as well as by fasting, yoga, and lying in the sun. Rejuvenation (*rasayana*) treatment is used to revitalize the body and can be performed by using various herbal preparations, medicated oil, and other agents such as certain metals. Mantras and meditations are also prescribed to improve spiritual well-being. Diet plays a vital role in the treatment regime.[4] A detailed discussion on Ayurveda is beyond the scope of this book, but we will look at common Ayurvedic medicines and their benefits and dangers.

TABLE 14.2: Cleansing Therapy (*Panchakarma*)

SANSKRIT NAME	WHAT IT MEANS
Basti	Enema
Nasya	Nasal administration of herbs such as sage, ginger, or calamus, or application of medicated oil in nasal passages
Rakta mokhsa	Release of toxic blood, not usually practiced today
Vamana	Therapeutic vomiting induced by herbs, salt, or emetics such as licorice
Virechan	Therapeutic purging using castor oil or senna

Ayurvedic Medicines

Ayurvedic treatment relies heavily on herbs, plant oils, and common spices. There are more than a thousand Ayurvedic formulas, and only a fraction of these have been investigated through the use of modern scientific methods. Ayurvedic medicines are composed of vegetables, animal products, minerals, spices, and herbal supplements. In the *Sushruta Samhita*, herbs have been classified into fifty groups according to their therapeutic actions. Minerals (gold, zinc, iron, copper, and mercury) are also used and are prepared as an ash (*bhasma*). The preparation of Ayurvedic medicines from bones and the flesh of goats, fish, and pecking birds, as well as aquatic and marshy animals, has been described in the *Sushruta Samhita*.[5] Common Ayurvedic medicines and their uses are listed in Table 14.3.

TABLE 14.3: Common Ayurvedic Medicines and Their Uses

Sanskrit Name	English Name	Use(s)
Ashwagandha	Winter cherry	Rejuvenating tonic
Amalaki, amla	Indian gooseberry	Antioxidant, antiaging
Atmagupta	Velvet bean	Anti-Parkinson's
Arjuna	n/a	Heart tonic, treating congestive heart failure
Bilva	Stone apple	Treating irritable bowel syndrome
Brahmi	n/a	Improving memory
Guggulu, guggul	Indian bdellium	Treating arthritis; improves lipid profile
Haridra	Turmeric	Improves lipid profile; may protect against Alzheimer's disease
Methika	Fenugreek	Treating diabetes and high lipids
Nimbo	Neem	Antibacterial, antifungal, antiviral
Mandukparni	Indian pennywort	Immune stimulant
Palandu	Onion	Improves lipid profile

Efficacy

Turmeric, derived from the plant *Curcuma longa,* is a popular Indian food condiment, and in Ayurvedic medicine it has been used for many centuries to treat a variety of conditions including pulmonary and gastrointestinal symptoms, skin rashes, sprains, wounds, and liver disease. Extensive scientific research in the past few decades has established that most activities of turmeric are due to its active ingredient, curcumin, which also gives turmeric its yellow color. Curcumin has been shown to have antioxidant, antibacterial, antifungal, antiviral, and anticancer activities.[6] Animal studies have shown that curcumin can reduce amyloid deposits in the brain and thus may be a very useful agent in treating Alzheimer's disease.[7]

I grew up in India, and my grandmother used to make a paste of turmeric with lime, heat it up, and apply it to any sprain I incurred from playing soccer. That paste worked like magic, and usually by the next morning I was pain-free. She also used lots of turmeric in cooking, and when my grandfather died at the age of eighty-eight and my grandmother died at the age of eighty-six, both had excellent mental clarity, never having suffered from age-related dementia. At our house in India we also had a tulsi plant (*Ocimum sanctum*), which many Indians consider holy. My grandmother used to make a paste from tulsi leaves and honey and give it to me when I got a cold or cough. The paste can be very helpful in alleviating the symptoms of colds or mild bronchial problems. Tulsi is an important plant in Ayurvedic medicine. Scientific studies have indicated analgesic, antifungal, and antibacterial effects.[8]

The neem tree (*Azadirachta indica*) is an important element in Ayurvedic medicine. All parts of the tree—leaves, flowers, seeds, fruits, and bark—have been used in traditional Ayurvedic medicine for treating inflammation, infection, fever, skin disease, and dental disorders. Neem toothpaste, prepared from neem extract, is a very popular brand in India and is also available in some Indian stores and health-food stores in the United States. It is believed that neem prevents cavity formation. Scientific research has demonstrated the anti-inflammatory, antimalarial, antifungal, antibacterial, antiviral, and anticancer activities of neem. Neem may also lower blood glucose.[9]

Several Ayurvedic herbal supplements such as ashwagandha, brahmi, mandukaparni, and sankhapuspi may improve memory and retard the brain-aging process.[10] Norh et al. studied the cholesterol-lowering effect of guggul, or guggulu, an herbal extract from the *Commiphora mukul* tree, and they observed that in thirty-four patients (eighteen taking guggul, sixteen taking placebo), after twelve weeks, the mean levels of cholesterol were reduced in the group who took guggul. However, the level of "bad" (low-density lipoprotein, or LDL) cholesterol and triglyceride concentrations did not change significantly between the two groups.[11] Many Ayurvedic medicines demonstrate excellent antioxidant properties.

Rigorous scientific research to evaluate the therapeutic benefits of Ayurvedic medicine is still in its early stages. Clinical trials showing the efficacy of a particular Ayurvedic formulation is often conducted with a limited number of subjects. The good news is that many Indian institutes, both governmental and nongovernmental, are actively undertaking research projects evaluating various Ayurvedic medicines and data is beginning to emerge on their efficacy and limitations. The Central Drug Research Institute in Lucknow, the National Institute of Ayurveda at Jaipur, and the Central Council for Research in Ayurveda and Siddha at New Delhi are a few examples of institutes in India where scientists are conducting rigorous research on Ayurvedic medicine.[12]

Dangers of Ayurvedic Medicines: Heavy-Metal Toxicity

In the United States, Ayurvedic medicines are considered dietary supplements and are sold under the Dietary Supplement Health and Education Act of 1994. As such, they are not required to meet the same rigorous standards as conventional medicines. Research has indicated that some Ayurvedic medicines contain heavy metals such as mercury, arsenic, and lead. In some of these medicines, metals are part of the formulation. *Bhasmas* are unique Ayurvedic metallic preparations containing herbal juices and fruits. They can be based on calcium, iron, zinc, mercury, silver, potassium, arsenic, copper, or tin, as well as on some gemstones. Trace amounts of gold can also be detected in some *bhasmas*. It is believed that metals exist as nanoparticles in *bhasmas*, are chelated with components of medicinal herbs, and are nontoxic. In siddha makaradhwaja, mercury is present as sulfide.[13] The basic materials of some Ayurvedic *bhasmas* are presented in Table 14.4, and although the basic materials of some *bhasmas* are not lead, arsenic, or copper, significant amounts of these metals may be found in these formulations.[14]

TABLE 14.4: Some Ayurvedic Medicines Containing Heavy Metals (*Bhasmas*)

BHASMA	BASIC MATERIAL*
Abrak	Manganese
Godanti	Gypsum
Loh	Iron
Mukta	Pearl
Naga	Lead
Parad	Mercury
Shanka	Seashells
Swarna	Gold
Trivang	Aluminum and zinc
Wang	Aluminum
Yased	Zinc

* Although arsenic, copper, or lead are not the basic ingredients of these *bhasmas*, significant amounts are found in these products.[15]

In 2004 Saper et al. published a paper in the *Journal of the American Medical Association* regarding the presence of heavy metals in some Ayurvedic herbal preparations available in the Boston area. The authors purchased Ayurvedic medicines from stores within a twenty-mile radius of Boston City Hall and, using a sophisticated technique called X-ray fluorescence spectroscopy, analyzed seventy of them for the presence of heavy metals. They observed that fourteen of the seventy herbal supplements analyzed (20 percent) contained heavy metals, including lead, mercury, and arsenic. Lead was found in thirteen preparations, mercury in six, and arsenic in six. The authors concluded that based on the amounts of heavy metals present in these supplements, if taken as recommended by the manufacturers, each of these fourteen preparations could result in heavy-metal intake above published regulatory limits and that users of Ayurvedic medicines might be at a risk for heavy-metal toxicity. The authors proposed that testing for heavy metals should be mandatory for Ayurvedic medicines.[16]

In a more recent study by Saper and his colleagues, 193 Ayurvedic medicines purchased from twenty-five websites of manufacturers from India and the United States were analyzed for the presence of heavy metals. As in their earlier studies, the authors observed that again 20.7 percent of all products contained heavy metals and approximately 80 percent did not. Of the U.S. products, 21 percent contained lead and 3 percent each contained mercury or arsenic. Among the Indian-made supplements, 17 percent contained lead, 7 percent contained mercury, and none contained arsenic. All metal-containing products exceeded one or more standards for acceptable daily intake of toxic metals. Among the metal-containing supplements, 75 percent of manufacturers claimed to have good manufacturing practices.[17] Table 14.5 presents a list of the medicines found to be tainted with heavy metals.

TABLE 14.5: Some Ayurvedic Medicines That Have Been Contaminated with Heavy Metals[18]

AYURVEDIC PRODUCT	MANUFACTURER	HEAVY METAL
Acnenil	Bazaar of India (U.S.)	Lead
Agnitundi Bati	Baidyanath Products (Indian)	Lead, mercury†
Amoebica	Baidyanath Products (Indian)	Lead
Arogyavardhini Bati	Baidyanath Products (Indian)	Lead, mercury†
Ayu Arthi-Tone	Sharangdhar Pharmaceuticals (Indian)	Lead
Ayu Hemoridi-Tone	Sharangdhar Pharmaceuticals (Indian)	Lead
Ayu Leuko-Tone	Sharangdhar Pharmaceuticals (Indian)	Lead
Ayu Nephro-Tone	Sharangdhar Pharmaceuticals (Indian)	Lead
AyurRelief	Balance Ayurvedic Products (U.S.)	Lead
Bacopa Monniera	Unknown (Indian)	Lead
Bakuchi	Bazaar of India (U.S.)	Lead
Brahmi	Baidyanath Products (Indian)	Lead
Brahmi	Bazaar of India (U.S.)	Lead

(cont'd.)

TABLE 14.5: Some Ayurvedic Medicines That Have Been Contaminated with Heavy Metals (cont'd)

AYURVEDIC PRODUCT	MANUFACTURER	HEAVY METAL
Chairata	Bazaar of India (U.S.)	Lead
Cold Aid	Bazaar of India (U.S.)	Lead
Commiphora Mukul	Unknown (Indian)	Mercury
Ekangvir Ras	Baidyanath Products (Indian)	Lead, mercury*
Energize	Bazaar of India (U.S.)	Lead
Ezi Slim	Goodcare Pharma (Indian)	Lead
GlucoRite	Balance Ayurvedic Products (U.S.)	Lead
Heart Plus	Bazaar of India (U.S.)	Lead
Hingwastika	Bazaar of India (U.S.)	Mercury
Jatamansi	Bazaar of India (U.S.)	Lead
Kanchanar Guggulu	Banyan Botanicals (U.S.)	Lead
Kanta Kari	Bazaar of India (U.S.)	Lead
Lean Plus	Tattva's Herbs (U.S.)	Lead
Licorice	Bazaar of India (U.S.)	Lead
Mahasudharshan	Banyan Botanicals (U.S.)	Lead
Neem	Tattva's Herbs (U.S.)	Lead
Prana—Breath of Life	Ayurherbal Corporation (U.S.)	Lead, mercury
Praval Pisti	Bazaar of India (U.S.)	Lead, mercury
Prostate Rejuv	Bazaar of India (U.S.)	Lead
Shilajit	Banyan Botanicals (U.S.)	Lead
Sugar Fight	Bazaar of India (U.S.)	Lead
Tagar	Bazaar of India (U.S.)	Lead
Trifala Guggulu	Bazaar of India (U.S.)	Arsenic, lead, mercury
Vital Lady	Maharishi Ayurveda (Indian)	Lead
Worry Free	Maharishi Ayurveda (Indian)	Lead
Yogaraj Guggulu	Unknown (Indian)	Mercury
Yograj Guggulu	Bazaar of India (U.S.)	Arsenic, lead

* Extremely high lead and mercury content

† Extremely high mercury content

Although approximately 95 percent of all lead poisoning among United States adults results from occupational exposure, consumption of Ayurvedic medicine contaminated with lead may also cause lead poisoning. During 2000–2003, a total of twelve cases of lead poisoning among adults in five states associated with consumption of Ayurvedic medicines were reported to the Centers for Disease

Control.[19] In a study by Kales et al., forty-seven published Ayurvedic heavy-metal poisoning cases (between 1996 and 2005) were analyzed. Four patients were seen at a referral center, and another nineteen patients with lead-paint intoxication were thoroughly analyzed. The authors observed that among the forty-seven patients with heavy-metal poisoning, coexposure to other metals was also common—23 percent of these patients were also exposed to arsenic. Arsenic is a known bone marrow toxin. Patients with lead poisoning due to the intake of Ayurvedic medicines often showed much higher blood lead levels compared with patients who experienced lead toxicity from exposure to lead-based paints. In addition, patients with lead poisoning related to the use of Ayurvedic medicines experienced more lead toxicity. One possible explanation is that individuals taking Ayurvedic medicines are not routinely evaluated for exposure to lead and seek medical attention only after clinical manifestation of lead toxicity.[20]

CASE STUDY

A thirty-seven-year-old man was admitted to the hospital due to weakness, dizziness, nausea, and muscle pain he had developed in the previous few weeks. A blood test indicated severe anemia with low hemoglobin, but thorough medical investigation did not identify any cause of anemia. At that point, the patient reported that he had traveled to India, where he visited an Ayurvedic practitioner who gave him several herbal remedies. He also received bowel washing with oil. He took most of these herbal remedies until a few days prior to his admission to the hospital. Lead poisoning was suspected, and his blood lead concentration was 38 mcg/100 mL, while normal level should be less than 10 mcg/100 mL. Analysis of the herbal supplement showed high lead content. The patient fully recovered after receiving chelation therapy with D-penicillamine.[21]

CASE STUDY

A thirty-five-year-old woman frequently visited the emergency room with severe colic pain, vomiting, and weight loss. Laboratory tests showed a low hemoglobin level, indicative of severe anemia. Examination of her blood cells (basophilic stripping in red blood cell smear) suggested lead poisoning, and her blood level of lead was elevated to a dangerous 140 mcg/100 mL. After ruling out all environmental exposure to lead, further investigation revealed that the woman was taking various Ayurvedic medicines. When those remedies were analyzed, one showed a high concentration of lead, and it was confirmed that her lead poisoning was due to ingestion of Ayurvedic medicine. The patient responded to chelation therapy and eventually recovered.[22]

A twenty-four-year-old pregnant woman who emigrated from India to Australia showed low hemoglobin at twenty-four weeks of pregnancy. Based on an analysis of her red blood cells (peripheral smear) her physician suspected lead poisoning, and it was found that she had a blood lead level of 107 mcg/100 mL, which was in the toxic range. Chelation therapy was initiated to treat her lead poisoning, and thirty-six hours later, the woman gave birth to a girl. The baby was critically ill and nonresponsive. Lead concentration in the cord blood was extremely high (157 mcg/100 mL), confirming severe lead poisoning in the newborn. Chelation therapy was initiated immediately, and the infant suffered for a long time due to maternal exposure to lead. At week fifteen, the blood level dropped to 37.2 mcg/100 mL and after five months to 19.5 mcg/100 mL. The source of the lead was confirmed as two Ayurvedic medicines the woman took periodically over a period of nine years following the recommendation of an Ayurvedic practitioner she visited in India. This case illustrates how lead poisoning in a mother can critically affect the health and well-being of her newborn.[23]

CASE STUDY

An eleven-year-old girl showed typical symptoms of arsenic toxicity and developed portal hypertension six months and eighteen months, respectively, after taking Ayurvedic medicines prescribed for epilepsy. Analysis of eight Ayurvedic medicines taken by the patient showed the presence of arsenic in the range of 5 mg/L to 248 mg/L (high), and her serum arsenic level was elevated to 202 mcg/L (normal is less than 60 mcg/L). After discontinuation of Ayurvedic medicines, her symptoms were resolved.[24]

CASE STUDY

Conclusion

The presence of lead and other heavy metals in Indian Ayurvedic medicines is due to multiple factors:

1. The heavy metal may be a part of the medicinal formula.

2. Environmental contamination is a major problem in India, and medicinal plants may be grown in urban areas where the soil is contaminated with heavy metals.

3. Manufacturing defects.

In general, Ayurvedic medicines prepared following the guidelines of *rasa shastra* contain higher amounts of metals compared with those not prepared this way. As a general practice, *rasa shastra* medicines contain various *bhasmas,* which contain high amounts of various metals. The proponents of this type of Ayurvedic medicine claim that if these metallic preparations were used with success for many centuries in India and if prepared following strict guidelines, then metal toxicity should not occur from using them because in the preparation phases metals undergo *shodona* (purification), in which their medicinal benefits are retained but their toxic properties are destroyed. These proponents blame heavy-metal toxicity from using these medicines to faulty industrial manufacturing processes and inadequate supervision of workers.[25]

Contamination of the irrigation water and soil in urban areas of India, where herbs used for manufacturing Ayurvedic medicines may be cultivated, is a problem. Although there is no published report of contamination of any herbal plant with heavy metals in India due to cultivation in contaminated soil, there are several reports of contaminated vegetables grown in soil containing heavy metals. Singh and Kumar reported that samples of spinach and okra grown in the outskirts of Delhi contained heavy metals such as zinc, lead, and cadmium at levels higher than permitted by the World Health Organization (WHO). Although amounts of heavy metals in soil where vegetables were grown were within permissible limits established by the WHO, they were higher in irrigation water.[26]

Regardless of the source of the heavy metals in some Ayurvedic medicine, using such medicines may put an individual at the risk of heavy-metal toxicity. Ayurvedic medicines prepared according to the formulas of *rasa shastra* should be avoided, and consultation with a knowledgeable Ayurvedic practitioner is essential if you wish to try any non-*rasa shastra* formula. In any case, it is essential that you tell your doctor if you are taking any Ayurvedic medicine so that proper blood tests can be ordered to determine your body's heavy-metal burden.

Unlike reports of adulteration of certain traditional medicines with pharmaceuticals, there is no report of adulteration of any Ayurvedic medicine with Western drugs. Therefore, the major danger at this point appears to be heavy-metal poisoning from a contaminated preparation.

Appendix A:
Generic and Trade Names of Drugs
Discussed in This Book

GENERIC NAME	REPRESENTATIVE TRADE NAME*
Analgesics	
Acetaminophen	Tylenol
Aspirin	Bayer, Bufferin
Diclofenac	Voltaren
Ibuprofen	Advil, Motrin
Indomethacin	Indocin
Mefenamic Acid	Ponstel
Naproxen	Aleve
Phenacetin	(Generic)
Tolmetin	Tolectin
Antiallergy drugs, cough suppressants	
Desloratadine	Clarinex
Dextromethorphan	Delsym, Robitussin Cough
Diphenhydramine	Benadryl
Fexofenadine	Allegra
Loratadine	Claritin
Terfenadine†	Seldane
Antiangina drugs	
Isosorbide	Isordil
Nifedipine	Procardia, Adalat
Nitroglycerin	Nitrospan, Nitrostat
Antianxiety drugs/Antidepressants	
Alprazolam	Xanax
Amitriptyline	Elavil
Clomipramine	Anafranil
Clonazepam	Klonopin
Chlordiazepoxide	Librium
Citalopram	Celexa
Desipramine	Norpramin
Diazepam	Valium

GENERIC NAME	REPRESENTATIVE TRADE NAME*
Fluoxetine	Prozac
Haloperidol	Haldol
Impramine	Tofranil
Lithium	Lithobid
Lorazepam	Ativan
Midazolam	Dormicum, Versed
Nefazodone	Nefadar
Paroxetine	Paxil
Phenelzine	Nardill
Sertraline	Zoloft
Trazodone	Desyrel
Triazolam	Halcion
Venlafaxine	Effexor
Mirtazapine	Remeron
Antiasthma drugs	
Theophylline	Aminophylline
Antibiotics/Anti-infectives	
Amikacin	Amikin
Amoxicillin	Amoxil
Ampicillin	Principen
Azithromycin	Zithromax
Cefuroxime	Ceftin
Ciprofloxacin	Cipro
Cycloserine	Seromycin
Doxycycline	Vibramycin
Erythromycin	E-Mycin
Gentamicin	Garamycin
Isoniazid	Nydrazid
Itraconazole	Sporanox
Ketoconazole	Nizoral
Metronidazole	Flagyl
Nitrofurantoin	Furadantin, Macrobid

(cont'd.)

Generic Name	Representative Trade Name*
Tetracycline	Achromycin V
Tinidazole	Tindamax
Vancomycin	Vancocin

Anticancer drugs

Generic Name	Representative Trade Name*
Imatinib	Gleevec
Irinotecan	Camptosar
Methotrexate	Rheumatrex
Paclitaxel	Taxol
Vinblastine	Velbe
Vincristine	Oncovin

Anticonvulsants

Generic Name	Representative Trade Name*
Carbamazepine	Tegretol
Phenytoin	Dilantin
Phenobarbital	Klonopin
Valproic acid	Depacon, Depakote

Antidiabetic drugs

Generic Name	Representative Trade Name*
Acetohexamide	Dymelor
Glibenclamide	Diabeta, Micronase
Gliclazide	Diamicron
Glyburide	Micronase
Metformin	Glucophage
Tolbutamide	Orinase

Antigout drugs

Generic Name	Representative Trade Name*
Allopurinal	Zyloprim

Antihypertensives

Generic Name	Representative Trade Name*
Benazepril	Lotensin
Clonidine	Catapres
Enalapril	Vaseretic
Felodipine	Plendil
Hydrochlorothiazide	(Generic)
Losartan	Cozaar
Nicardipine	Cardene
Nisoldipine	Sular
Nitrendipine	Cardif, Nitrepin
Pranidipine	Acalas
Prazosin	Minipress
Propanolol	Inderal
Quinapril	Accupril
Terazosin	Hytrin

Anti-HIV drugs

Generic Name	Representative Trade Name*
Saquinavir	Invirase, Fortovase
Alazanavir	Reyataz
Lamivudine	Epivir, Zeffix
Zidovudine (AZT)	Retrovir
Indinavir	Crixivan
Ritonavir	Norvir
Nevirapine	Viramune

Antimalarials

Generic Name	Representative Trade Name*
Chloroquine	Aralen

Anti-Parkinson's drugs

Generic Name	Representative Trade Name*
Levodopa	Dopar, Larodopa

Antivirals

Generic Name	Representative Trade Name*
Foscanet	Foscavin

Bloot clot–prevention drugs

Generic Name	Representative Trade Name*
Warfarin	Coumadin

Cardioactive drugs

Generic Name	Representative Trade Name*
Amiodarone	Cordarone, Pacerone
Digoxin	Lanoxin
Lovastatin	Altocor, Mevacor
Propanolol	Inderal
Quinidine	Quinaglute
Verapamil	Calan, Isoptin, Verelan

Cholesterol-lowering drugs

Generic Name	Representative Trade Name*
Atorvastatin	Lipitor
Niacin	Niaspan
Pravastatin	Pravachol
Pravastatin + aspirin	Pravigard
Simvastatin	Zocor

Erectile-dysfunction drugs

Generic Name	Representative Trade Name*
Sildenafil	Viagra

Heartburn drugs/acid-reflux relievers

Generic Name	Representative Trade Name*
Cimetidine	Tagamet
Ranitidine	Zantac
Metoclopramide	Reglan
Nizatidine	Axid

(cont'd.)

Generic Name	Representative Trade Name*
Immunosuppressants	
Tacrolimus	Prograf
Cyclosporine	Neoral, Sandimmune
Mycophenolic acid	CellCept
Muscle-pain relievers	
Cyclobenzaprine	Flexeril
Carisoprodol	Soma
Muscle relaxants	
Chlorzoxazone	Anectine, Scoline
Suxamethonium	Paraflex
Sedatives	
Pentobarbital	Nembutal
Severe-pain relievers	
Hydrocodone/ acetiminophen	Vicodin

* There may be multiple trade names of a drug manufactured by different pharmaceutic companies.

† Withdrawn from the market.

Generic Name	Representative Trade Name*
Meperidine	Demerol
Oxycodone/ acetaminophen	Percocet
Propoxyphene/ acetaminophen	Darvocet-N
Sleeping aids	
Diphenhydramine	Benadryl
Doxylamine	Unisom
Estazolam	ProSom
Temazepam	Restoril
Zolpidem	Ambien
Steroids	
Clobetasol propionate	Clobex
Dexamethasone	Dexacort
Fluocinolone	Fluonid, Synemol
Hydrocortisone	Cortizone, Hydro-cortone
Prednisolone	Prelone, Econopred

Appendix B:
Herbal Supplements You Should Avoid
Because They Are Potentially Toxic

The following list of herbal supplements that are advisable to avoid is probably conservative, but it is better to be safe than sorry. Other herbs may also have adverse effects on humans. This list is not complete but covers commonly encountered, relatively toxic, herbs.

- bitter orange
- calamus
- chaparral
- Chinese herbs containing aristolochic acid
- coltsfoot
- ephedra
- guarana
- kombucha mushroom
- mistletoe
- pennyroyal
- skullcap
- wormwood
- borage
- Chan Su
- Chinese herbs containing aconite
- comfrey
- germander
- kava
- lobelia
- oleander
- pokeweed
- thunder-god vine
- yohimbe

Notes

Chapter 1: Complementary and Alternative Medicines: Who Uses Them?

1. J.L. Swerdlow, "Medicine Changes: Late 19th to Early 20th Century," in *Nature's Medicines: Plants That Heal* (Washington, D.C.: National Geographic Society, 2000): 158–91.

2. T.B. Klepser, "Unsafe and Potentially Safe Herbal Therapies," *American Journal of Health–System Pharmacy* 56 (1999): 125–41.

3. E. Mills et al., "Impact of Federal Safety Advisories on Health Food Store Advice," *Journal of General Internal Medicine* 19 (2004): 269–72.

4. G. Calapai, "European Legislation on Herbal Medicines: A Look into the Future," *Drug Safety* 31 (2008): 428–31.

5. K. Moss et al., "New Canadian Natural Health Product Regulations: A Qualitative Study on How CAM Practitioners Perceive They Will Be Impacted," *BMC Complementary and Alternative Medicine* 10, no. 6 (2006): 18.

6. J.P. Kelly et al., "Recent Trends in Use of Herbal and Other Natural Products," *Archives of Internal Medicine* 165 (2005): 281–86.

7. G.B. Mahady, "Global Harmonization of Herbal Health Claims," *Journal of Nutrition* 131 (2001): 1120S–23S.

8. S. Bent, "Herbal Medicine in the United States: Review of Efficacy, Safety and Regulation," *Journal of General Internal Medicine* 23 (2008): 854–59.

9. J.I. Mechanick, "The Rational Rise of Dietary Supplements and Neutraceuticals in Clinical Medicine," *Mount Sinai Journal of Medicine* 72 (2005): 161–65.

10. H. Ni, C. Simile, and A.M. Hardy, "Utilization of Complementary and Alternative Medicine by United States Adults," *Medical Care* 40 (2002): 353–58; H.A. Tindle et al., "Trends in Use of Complementary and Alternative Medicine by U.S. Adults 1997–2002," *Alternative Therapies in Health and Medicine* 11 (2005): 42–49.

11. Tindle et al., "Trends in Use," 42–49.

12. Ni, Simile, and Hardy, "Utilization of Complementary," 353–58.

13. Tindle et al., "Trends in Use," 42–49.

14. A. Vitale, "An Integrative Review of Reiki Touch Therapy Research," *Holistic Nursing Practice* 21 (2007): 169–79.

15. C.D. Myers, T. Walton, and B.J. Small, "The Value of Massage Therapy in Cancer Care," *Hematology/Oncology Clinics of North America* 22 (2008): 649–60.

16. L. Esmond and A.R.F. Long, "Complementary Therapy Use by Persons with Multiple Sclerosis: Benefits and Research Priorities," *Complementary Therapies in Clinical Practice* 14 (2008): 176–84.

17. F. Quinn, C.M. Huges, and G.D. Baxter, "Reflexology in the Management of Low Back Pain: A Pilot Randomized Controlled Trial," *Complementary Therapies in Clinical Practice* 16 (2008): 3–8.

18. N.S. Gooneratne, "Complementary and Alternative Medicine for Sleep Disturbances in Older Adults," *Clinics in Geriatric Medicine* 24 (2008): 121–38.

19. S. Birch et al., "Clinical Research on Acupuncture, Part 1: What Have Reviews of the Efficacy and Safety of Acupuncture Told Us So Far?" *Journal of Alternative and Complementary Medicine* 10 (2004): 468–80.

20. E. Manheimer et al., "Meta-Analysis: Acupuncture for Low Back Pain," *Annals of Internal Medicine* 142 (2005): 651–63.

21. X.Y. Wang et al., "Abdominal Acupuncture for Insomnia in Women: A Randomized Controlled Study," *Acupuncture Electrotherapy Research* 33 (2008): 33–41.

22. G.S. Bridee et al., "Characteristics of Yoga Users: Results of a National Survey," *Journal of General Internal Medicine* 10 (2008): 1653–58.

23. P.R. Pullen et al., "Effects of Yoga on Inflammation and Exercise Capacity in Patients with Chronic Heart Failure," *Journal of Cardiac Failure* 14 (2008): 407–13.

24. S.R. Jayasinghe, "Yoga in Cardiac Health (a Review)," *European Journal of Cardiovascular Prevention and Rehabilitation* 11 (2004): 369–75.

25. K.Y. Fong et al., "Basilar Artery Occlusion Following Yoga Exercise," *Clinical and Experimental Neurology* 30 (1993): 104–9.

26. A.J. Araisa et al., "Systematic Review of Efficacy of Meditation Techniques as Treatments for Medical Illness," *Journal of Alternative and Complementary Medicine* 12 (2006): 817–32.

27. P.S. Mueller, D.J. Plevak, and T.A. Rummans, "Religious Involvement, Spirituality and Medicine: Implications for Clinical Practice," *Mayo Clinic Proceedings* 76 (2001): 1225–35.

28. S. Cotton et al., "Religion/Spirituality and Adolescent Health Outcome: A Review," *Journal of Adolescent Health* 38 (2006): 472–80.

29. M. Meraviglia, "Effects of Spirituality in Breast Cancer Survivors," *Oncology Nursing Forum* 33 (2006): E1–7.

30. Tindle et al., "Trends in Use," 42–49.

31. Ni, Simile, and Hardy, "Utilization of Complementary," 353–58.

32. M.J. Tanaka et al., "Patterns of Natural Herb Use by Asian and Pacific Islanders," *Ethnicity & Health* 13 (2008): 93–108.

33. J. Duggan et al., "Use of Complementary and Alternative Therapies in HIV-Infected Patients," *AIDS Patient Care and STDs* 15 (2001): 159–67.

34. A. Owen-Smith, R. Diclemente, and G. Wingood, "Complementary and Alternative Medicine Use Decreases Adherence to HAART in HIV-Positive Women," *AIDS Care* 19 (2007): 589–93.

35. J.W. Henderson and R.J. Donatelle, "Complementary and Alternative Medicine Use by Women after Completion of Allopathic Treatment for Breast Cancer," *Alternative Therapies in Health and Medicine* 10 (2004): 52–57.

36. P. Gardiner et al., "Herb Use Among Health Care Professionals Enrolled in an Online Curriculum on Herbs and Dietary Supplements," *Journal of Herbal Pharmacotherapy* 6 (2006): 51–64.

37. P. Gardiner, et al., "Factors Associated with Herbal Therapy Use by Adults in the United States," *Alternative Therapies in Health and Medicine* 13 (2007): 22–28.

38. P. Gardiner et al., "Factors Associated with Dietary Supplement Use Among Prescription Medication Users," *Archives of Internal Medicine* 166 (2006): 1968–74.

39. L.J. Standish et al., "Alternative Medicine Use in HIV Positive Men and Women: Demographics, Utilization Patterns and Health Status," *AIDS Care* 13 (2001): 197–208.

Chapter 2: Some Relatively Safe and Effective Herbal Supplements

1. P. Gardiner et al., "Factors Associated with Herbal Therapy Use by Adults in the United States," *Alternative Therapies in Health and Medicine* 13 (2007): 22–29.

2. B.A. Messina, "Herbal Supplements: Facts and Myths—Talking to Your Patients About Herbal Supplements," *Journal of PeriAnesthesia Nursing* 21 (2006): 268–78.

3. R. Maenthaisong et al., "The Efficacy of Aloe Vera Used for Burn Wound Healing: A Systematic Review," *Burns* 33 (2007): 713–18.

4. L. Langmed et al., "Randomized Double-Blind Placebo-Controlled Trial of Oral Aloe Vera Gel for Active Ulcerative Colitis," *Ailment Pharmacology and Therapeutics* 19 (2004): 739–47.

5. Ibid.

6. M. Prichard and K.J. Turner, "Acute Hypersensitivity to Ingested Processed Pollen," *Aust N Z J med* 15 (1985): 346–47.

7. S. Zafra-Stones et al., "Berry Anthrocyanins as Novel Antioxidants in Human Health and Disease Prevention," *Molecular Nutrition and Food Research* 51 (2007): 675–83.

8. S.R. Hardin, "Cat's Claw: An Amazonian Vine Decreases Inflammation in Osteoarthritis," *Complementary Therapies in Clinical Practice* 2007; 13: 25–28.

9. M. O'Hara et al., "A Review of 12 Commonly Used Medicinal Herbs," *Archives of Family Medicine* 7 (1998): 523–36.

10. R. Award et al., "Effects of Traditionally Used Anxiolytic Botanicals on Enzymes of the Gamma-Aminobutyric (GABA) System," *Canadian Journal of Physiology and Pharmacology* 85(2007): 933–42.

11. K. Schütz, R. Carle, and A. Schieber, "Taraxacum—A Review on Its Phytochemical and Pharmacological Profile," *Journal of Ethnopharmacology* 107 (2006): 313–23.

12. A. Basch et al., "Therapeutic Applications of Fenugreek," *Alternative Medicine Review* 8 (2003): 20–27.

13. J.A. Abdel-Barry et al., "Hypoglycemic Effect of Aqueous Extract of Leaves of *Trigonella Foenum* in Healthy Volunteers," *Eastern Mediterranean Health Journal* 6 (2000): 83–88.

14. Basch et al., "Therapeutic Applications," 20–27.

15. R.J. Marle, J. Kaminski, and J.T. Arnason, "A Bioassay for the Inhibition of Serotonin Release from Bovine Platelets," *Journal of Natural Products* 55 (1992): 1044–56.

16. E.S. Johnson, "Efficacy of Feverfew as a Prophylactic Treatment of Migraine," *British Medical Journal* 291 (1985): 569–73.

17. J.J. Murphy, S. Heptinstall, and J.R.A. Mitchell, "Randomised Double-Blind Placebo-Controlled Trial of Feverfew in Migraine Prevention," *Lancet* 2 (1988): 189–92.

18. M. Schurks, H.C. Diener, and P. Goadsby, "Update on the Prophylaxis of Migraine," *Current Treatment Options in Neurology* 10 (2008): 20–29.

19. W. Abebe, "Herbal Medications: Potential for Adverse Interactions with Analgesic Drugs," *Journal of Clinical Pharmacy and Therapeutics* 27 (2002): 391–401.

20. E.A. Lucas et al., "Flaxseed Improved Lipid Profile Without Altering Biomarkers of Bone Metabolism in Postmenopausal Women," *Journal of Clinical Endocrinology and Metabolism* 87 (2002): 1527–32.

21. O'Hara et al., "Review of 12," 523–36.

22. D.L. Morse et al., "Garlic-in-Oil Associated Botulism: Episode Leads to Product Modification," *American Journal of Public Health* 80 (1990): 1272–1373.

23. S. Phillips, R. Ruggier, and S.E. Hutchinson, "*Zingiber Officinale* (Ginger): An Anti-emetic for Day Care Surgery," *Anesthesia* 48 (1993): 715–17.

24. A. Wettstein, "Cholinesterase Inhibitors and Ginkgo Extracts—Are They Comparable in Treatment of Dementia? Comparison of Published Placebo-Controlled Efficacy of at Least Six Months' Duration," *Phytomedicine* 6 (2000): 393–401.

25. H. Allain et al., "Effect of Two Doses of Ginkgo Biloba Extract (Egb 761) on Dual-Coding Test in Elderly Subjects," *Clinical Therapeutics* 15 (1993): 549–57.

26. S.T. DeKosky et al., "Ginkgo Biloba for Prevention of Dementia: A Randomized Controlled Trial," *Journal of the American Medical Association* 300 (2008): 2253–62.

27. G.J. Gilbert, "Ginkgo Biloba," *Neurology* 48 (1997): 1137.

28. M. Rosenblatt and J. Mindel, "Spontaneous Hyphema Associated with Ingestion of Ginkgo Biloba Extract," *New England Journal of Medicine* 336 (1997): 1108.

29. O'Hara et al., "Review of 12," 523–36.

30. Ibid.

31. R. Siegal, "Ginseng Abuse Syndrome: Problems with the Panacea," *Journal of the American Medical Association* 241 (1979): 1614–15.

32. D. Bagchi et al., "Molecular Mechanisms of Cardioprotection by a Novel Grape Seed Proanthocyanidin Extract," *Mutation Research* 523–24 (2003): 87–97.

33. H. Fujiki, "Green Tea: Health Benefits as Cancer Preventive for Humans," *Chemical Research* 5 (2005): 119–32.

34. D.J. Maron et al., "Cholesterol-Lowering Effect of a Theaflavin-Enriched Green Tea Extract: A Randomized Controlled Trial," *Archives of Internal Medicine* 163 (2003): 1448–1553.

35. P. Auvichayapat et al., "Effectiveness of Green Tea on Weight Reduction in Obese Thais: A Randomized, Controlled Trial," *Physiology and Behavior* 93 (2008): 486–91.

36. M.H. Pittler, R. Guo, and E. Ernst, "Hawthorn Extract for Treating Chronic Heart Failure," *Cochrane Database Systematic Review* 23 (2008): CD005312.

37. M.H. Pittler and E. Ernst, "Horse-Chestnut Seed Extract for Chronic Venous Insufficiency: A Criteria-Based Systematic Review," *Archives of Dermatology* 134 (1998): 1356–60.

38. C.R. Sirtori, "Aescin: Pharmacology, Pharmacokinetics and Therapeutic Profile," *Pharmacological Research* 44 (2001): 183–93.

39. R.A. Isbrucker and G.A. Buedock, "Risk and Assessment on the Consumption of Licorice Root (*Glycyrrhiza sp*), Its Extract and Powder As a Food Ingredient with

Emphasis on the Pharmacology and Toxicology of Glycyrrhizin," *Regulation Toxicology and Pharmacology* 46 (2006): 167–92.

40. C. Fiore et al., "Antiviral Effects of Glycyrrhiza Species," *Phytotherapy Research* 22 (2008): 141–48.

41. W. Najim and D.L. Lie, "Dietary Supplements Commonly Used for Prevention," *Primary Care Clinical Office Practice* 35 (2008): 749–67.

42. Ibid.

43. O'Hara et al., "Review of 12," 523–36.

44. F. Rainone, "Milk Thistle," *American Family Physician* 72 (2005): 1285–88.

45. C. Tamayo and S. Diamond, "Review of Clinical Trials Evaluating Safety and Efficacy of Milk Thistle (*Silybum marianum* [L] Gaertn)," *Integrative Cancer Therapies* 6 (2007): 146–57.

46. M. Wang et al., "*Morinda citrifolia* (Noni): A Literature Review and Recent Advances in Noni Research," *Acta Pharmacologica Sinica* 23 (2002): 1127–41.

47. V. Stadlbauer et al., "Hepatotoxicity of Noni Juice: Report of Two Cases," *World Journal of Gastroenterology* 11 (2005): 4758–60.

48. J.C. Carraro, J.P. Raynaud, and G. Koch, "Comparison of Phytotherapy (Permixon) with Finasteride in the Treatment of Benign Prostate Hyperplasia: A Randomized International Study of 1,098 Patients," *Prostate* 29 (1996): 231–40.

49. L.S. Marks et al., "Effects of Saw Palmetto Herbal Blend in Men with Symptomatic Benign Prostatic Hyperplasia," *Journal of Urology* 163 (2000): 1451–56.

50. B. Vanderperren et al., "Acute Liver Failure with Renal Impairment Related to the Abuse of Senna Anthraquinone Glycoside," *Annals of Pharmacotherapy* 39 (2005): 1353–57.

51. M.T. Velasquez and S.J. Bhathena, "Role of Dietary Soy in Obesity," *International Journal of Medical Sciences* 26 (2007): 72–82.

52. C.R. Sirtori and M.R. Lovati, "Soy Proteins and Cardiovascular Disease," *Current Atherosclerosis Report* 3 (2001): 47–53.

53. M.S. Kurzer, "Soy Consumption for Reduction of Menopausal Symptoms," *Inflammopharmacology* 16 (2008): 227–29.

54. K. Linde et al., "St. John's Wort for Depression: An Overview and Meta-Analysis of Randomised Clinical Trials," *British Medical Journal* 313 (1996): 253–58.

55. S. Kasper et al, "Efficacy of St. John's Wort Extract WS 5570 in Acute Treatment of Mild Depression: A Reanalysis of Data from Controlled Clinical Trials," *European Archives of Psychiatry and Clinical Neuroscience* 258 (2008): 59–63.

56. G.M. Bove, "Acute Neuropathy After Exposure to Sun in a Patient Treated with St. John's Wort," *Lancet* 352 (1998): 1121–22.

57. B.B. Aggarwal et al., "Curcumin: The Indian Solid Gold," *Advances in Experimental Medicine and Biology* 595 (2007): 1–75.

58. J.L. Funk et al., "Turmeric Extracts Containing Curcuminoids Prevent Experimental Rheumatoid Arthritis," *Journal of Natural Products* 69 (2006): 351–55.

59. P.D. Leathwood et al., "Aqueous Extract of Valerian Root (*Valeriana officinalis L*) Improves Sleep Quality in Man," *Pharmacol Biochemistry and Behavior* 17 (1982): 65–71.

60. A. Brattstrom, "Scientific Evidence for a Fixed Extract Combination (Ze01019) from Valerian and Hops Traditionally Used As a Sleep Inducing Aid," *Wiener Medizinische Wochenschrift* 157 (2007): 367–70.

61. A.J. Wagernmakers, "Amino Acid Supplements to Improve Athletic Performance," *Current Opinion in Clinical Nutrition and Metabolic Care* 2, no. 6 (1999): 539–44.

62. R.A. Bonakdar and E. Guarneri, "Coenzyme Q10," *American Family Physician* 72 (2005): 1065–70.

63. S. Pepe et al., "Coenzyme Q10 in Cardiovascular Disease," *Mitochondrion* 7 Suppl (June 2007): S154–67.

64. T.W. Demant and E.C. Rhodes, "Effects of Creatine Supplementation on Exercise Performance," *Sports Medicine* 28 (1999): 49–60.

65. D.R. Cameron and G.D. Braunstein, "The Use of Dehydroepiandrosterone Therapy in a Clinical Practice," *Treatment in Endocrinology* 4 (2005): 95–114.

66. Najim and Lie, "Dietary Supplements Commonly Used," 749–67.

67. S. Russell, "Carnitine as an Antidote for Acute Valproate Toxicity in Children," *Current Opinion in Pediatrics* 19 (2007): 206–10.

68. A. Herxheimer and K.J. Petrie, "Melatonin for the Prevention and Treatment of Jet Lag," *Cochrane Database Systematic Review* 1 (2002): CD001520.

69. B. Poeggeler, "Melatonin, Aging, and Age-Related Diseases: Perspectives for Prevention, Intervention, and Therapy," *Endocrine* 27 (2005): 201–12.

70. Najim and Lie, "Dietary Supplements Commonly Used," 749–67.

71. R.B. Saper, D.M. Eisenberg, and R.S. Phillips, "Common Dietary Supplements for Weight Loss," *American Family Physician* 70 (2004): 1731–38.

Chapter 3: Essential Oils and Fish-Oil Supplements: How Effective Are They?

1. A.E. Edris, "Pharmaceutical and Therapeutic Potential of Essential Oils and Their Individual Volatile Constituents: A Review," *Phytotherapy Research* 21 (2007): 308–21.

2. N. Perry and E. Perry, "Aromatherapy in the Management of Psychiatric Disorders: Clinical and Neuropharmacological Perspectives," *CNS Drugs* 20 (2006): 257–80.

3. D.M. Reith, W.R. Pitt, and R. Hockey, "Childhood Poisoning in Queensland: An Analysis of Presentation and Admission Rate," *Journal of Paediatrics & Child Health* 37 (2001): 262–65.

4. M. Botma, W. Colquhoun-Flannery, and S. Leighton, "Laryngeal Edema Caused by Accidental Ingestion of Oil of Wintergreen," *International Journal of Pediatric Otorhinolaryngology* 58 (2001): 229–32.

5. S.E. Janes and C.S.G. Price, "Essential Oil Poisoning: N-Acetylcysteine for Eugenol Induced Hepatic Failure and Analysis of a National Database," *European Journal of Pediatrics* 164 (2005): 520–522.

6. M.C. Morris, A. Donoghue, J.A. Markowitz, and K.C. Osterhoudt, "Ingestion of Tea Tree Oil (Melaleuca Oil) by a 4-Year-Old Boy," *Pediatric Emergency Care* 19 (2003): 169–71.

7. M. Nagamura, S. Hirose, Y. Nakayama, and K. Nakajima, "A Study of the Phototoxicity of Lemon Oil," *Archives of Dermatological Research* 278 (1985): 31–36.

8. S. Kaddu, H. Kerl, and P. Wolf, "Accidental Bullous Phototoxic Reactions to Bergamot Aromatherapy Oil," *Journal of the American Academy of Dermatology* 45 (2001): 458–61.

9. S. Prabuseenivasan, M. Jayakumar, and S. Ignacimuthu, "In Vitro Antibacterial Activity of Some Plant Essential Oils," *BMC Complementary and Alternative Medicine* 30, no. 6 (2006): 39.

10. B. Ouattara et al., "Antibacterial Activity of Selected Fatty Acids of Essential Oils Against Six Meat Spoilage Organisms," *Internation Journal of Food Microbiology* 37 (1997): 155–62.

11. V. Calabrese, S.D. Randazzo, C. Catalano, and V. Rizza, "Biochemical Study on a Novel Antioxidant from Lemon Oil and its Biotechnological Application in Cosmetic Dermatology," *Drugs Under Experimental and Clinical Research* 25 (1999): 219–225.

12. Prabuseenivasan, Jayakumar, and Ignacimuthu, "In Vitro Antibacterial Activity," 39.

13. L. Hagvall et al., "Lavender Oil Lacks Natural Protection Against Autoxidation, Forming Strong Contact Allergens on Air Exposure," *Contact Dermatitis* 59 (2008): 143–50.

14. C. Crason and T. Riley, "Toxicity of Essential Oil of *Melaleuca Alternifolia* or Tea Tree Oil," *Clinical Toxicology* 33 (1995): 193–95.

15. J. Reichiling et al., "Topical Tea Tree Oil Effective in Canine Localized Pruritic Dermatitis—A Multicenter Randomized Double-Blind Controlled Clinical Trial in the Veterinary Practice," *Deutsch Tierarztlichel Wochenschrift* 111 (2004): 408–414.

16. Prabuseenivasan, Jayakumar, and Ignacimuthu, "In Vitro Antibacterial Activity," 39.

17. C.H. Charles et al., "Comparative Antiplaque and Antigingivitis Effectiveness of a Chlorhexidine and an Essential Oil Mouthrinse: 6-Month Clinical Trial," *Journal of Clinical Periodontology* 31 (2004): 878–84.

18. I. Rasooli, S. Shayegh, M. Taghizadeh, and S.D. Astaneh, "Phytotherapy Prevention of Dental Biofilm Formation," *Phytotherapy Research* 22 (2008): 1162–67.

19. Prabuseenivasan, Jayakumar, and Ignacimuthu, "In Vitro Antibacterial Activity," 39.

20. J. Gutierrez, C. Barry-Ryan, and P. Bourke, "The Antimicrobial Efficacy of Plant Essential Oil Combinations and Infections with Food Ingredients," *International Journal of Food Microbiology* 124 (2008): 91–97.

21. J. Gutierrez, G. Rodriguez, C. Barry-Ryan, and P. Bourke, "Efficacy of Plant Essential Oils Against Food-Borne Pathogens and Spoilage Bacteria Associated with Ready-to-Eat Vegetables: Antimicrobial and Sensory Screening," *Journal of Food Protection* 71 (2008): 1846–1854.

22. Prabuseenivasan, Jayakumar, and Ignacimuthu, "In Vitro Antibacterial Activity," 39.

23. C. Koch et al., "Efficacy of Anise Oil, Dwarf Pine Oil and Chamomile Oil Against Thymidine-Kinase Positive and Thymidine-Kinase Negative Herpesvirus," *Journal of Pharmacy and Pharmacology* 60 (2008): 1545–50.

24. Prabuseenivasan, Jayakumar, and Ignacimuthu, "In Vitro Antibacterial Activity," 39.

25. A. Wei and T. Shibamoto, "Antioxidant Activities and Volatile Constituents of Various Essential Oils," *Journal of Agricultural and Food Chemistry* 55 (2007): 1737–42.

26. Perry and Perry, "Aromatherapy in the Management," 257–280.

27. J. Henry et al., "Lavender for Night Sedation of People with Dementia," *International Journal of Aromatherapy* 5 (1994): 28–30.

28. M.C. Beshara and D. Giddings, "Use of Plant Essential Oils in Treating Agitation in a Dementia Unit: 10 Case Studies," *International Journal of Aromatherapy* 12 (2003): 207–12.

29. Perry and Perry, "Aromatherapy in the Management," 257–280.

30. Prabuseenivasan, Jayakumar, and Ignacimuthu, "In Vitro Antibacterial Activity," 39.

31. K.M. Reinhart, C.I. Coleman, C. Teevan, and P. Vachhani, "Effects of Garlic on Blood Pressure in Patients with and without Systolic Hypertension: A Meta Analysis," *Annals of Pharmacotherapy* 42 (2008): 1766–71.

32. Prabuseenivasan, Jayakumar, and Ignacimuthu, "In Vitro Antibacterial Activity," 39.

33. Y.B. Yip and A.C. Tam, "An Experimental Study on the Effectiveness of Massage with Aromatic Ginger and Orange Essential Oil for Moderate to Severe Knee Pain Among the Elderly in Hong Kong," *Complementary Therapies in Medicine* 16 (2008): 131–38.

34. A. Woolf, "Essential Oil Poisoning," *Journal of Toxicology: Clinical Toxicology* 37 (1999): 721–27.

35. Janes and Price, "Essential Oil Poisoning," 520–522.

36. H.O. Bang, J. Dyreberg, and N. Hjoome, "The Composition of Food Consumed by Greenland Eskimos," *Acta Medica Scandanavia* 200 (1976): 69–73.

37. H. Leon et al., "Effect of Fish Oil on Arrhythmias and Mortality: Systematic Review," *British Medical Journal* 23 (2008): 337: a2931.

38. American Heart Association, "Fish and Omega-3 Fatty Acids." (http://american heart.org/presenter.jhtml?identifier=4632). Accessed 11 January 2009.

39. S.M. Proudman, L.G. Cleland, and M.J. James, "Dietary Omega-3 Fats for Treatment of Inflammatory Joint Disease: Efficacy and Utility," *Rheumatic Disease Clinics of North America* 34 (2008): 469–79.

40. M.S. Buckley, A.D. Goff, and W.E. Knapp, "Fish Oil Interaction with Warfarin," *Annals of Pharmacotherapy* 38 (2004): 50–52.

41. American Heart Association, "Fish and Omega-3 Fatty Acids."

42. H.E. Bayes, "Safety Considerations with Omega-3 Fatty Acid Therapy," *American Journal of Cardiology* 99 (2007): 35C–43C.

Chapter 4: Herbal Supplements That May Boost Your Immune System

1. M. Roxas and J. Jurenka, "Colds and Influenza: A Review of Diagnosis and Conventional Botanicals, and Nutritional Considerations," *Alternative Medicine Review* 12 (2007): 25–48.

2. W.C. Cho and K.N. Leung, "In Vitro and In Vivo Immunomodulating and Immunorestorative Effects of Astragalus Membranaceus," *Journal of Ethnopharmacology* 113 (2007): 132–41.

3. Z.G. Liu, Z.M. Xiong, and X.Y. Yu, "Effect of Astragalus Injection on Immune Function in Patients with Congestive Heart Failure," *Zhongguo Zhong Xi Yi Jie He Za Zhi* 23 (2003): 351–53.

4. K.K. Auyeung, P.C. Law, and J.K. Ko, "Astragalus Saponins Induce Apoptosis via an ERK-Independent NF-Kappa B Signaling Pathway in Human Hepatocellular HepG2 Cell Line," *International Journal of Molecular Medicine* 23 (2009): 189–96.

5. B. Leutting et al., "Macrophage Activation by the Polysaccharide Arabinogalactan Isolated from Plant Cell Culture of *Echinacea Purpurea*," *Journal of the National Cancer Institute* 81 (1989): 669–75.

6. S.A. Hwang, A. Dasgupta, and J.K. Actor, "Cytokine Production by Non-Adherent Mouse Splenocyte Cultures to Echinacea Extracts," *Clinica Chimica Acta* 343 (2004): 161–66.

7. A.M. Sullivan, J.G. Laba, J.A. Moore, and T.D. Lee, "Echinacea-Induced Macrophage Activation," *Immunopharmacology and Immunotoxicology* 30 (2008): 553–74.

8. W.E. Melchart, K. Linde, R. Brandmaier, and C. Lersch, "Echinacea Root Extracts for the Prevention of Upper Respiratory Tract Infection: A Double-Blind, Placebo-Controlled Randomized Trial," *Archives of Family Medicine* 7 (1998): 541–45.

9. R. Schoop, P. Klein, A. Suter, and S.L. Johnston, "Echinacea in the Prevention of Induced Rhinovirus Colds: A Meta-Analysis," *Clinical Therapeutics* 28 (2006): 174–83.

10. A.L. Huntley, J. Thompson Coon, and E. Ernst, "The Safety of Herbal Medicinal Products Derived From Echinacea Species: A Systematic Review," *Drug Safety* 28 (2005): 387–400.

11. Z. Zakay-Rines, E. Thom, T. Wollen, and J. Wadstein, "Randomized Study of the Efficacy and Safety of Oral Elderberry Extract in the Treatment of Influenza A and B," *Journal of International Medical Research* 32 (2004): 132–40.

12. A. Serafino et al., "Stimulatory Effect of Eucalyptus Essential Oil on Innate Cell Mediated Immune Response," *BMC Immunology* 18, no. 9 (2008): 17.

13. H. Amagase, "Clarifying the Real Bioactive Constituents of Garlic," *Journal of Nutrition* 136, suppl. 3 (2006): 716–25.

14. P. Josling, "Preventing the Common Cold with a Garlic Supplement: A Double-blind Study," *Advances in Therapeutics* 18, no. 4 (2001): 189–93.

15. D. Kiefer and T. Pantuso, "Panax ginseng," *American Family Physician* 68 (2003): 1539–42.

16. G.N. Predy et al., "Efficacy of an Extract of North American Ginseng Containing Poly-Furanosyl-Pyranosyl-Saccharides for Preventing Upper Respiratory Tract Infections: A Randomized Controlled Trial," *Canadian Medical Association Journal* 173 (2005): 1043–48.

17. T.S. Kim et al., "Induction of Interleukin 12 Production in Mouse Macrophages by Berberine, a Benzodioxoloquinolizine Alkaloid Deviates CD+ T cells from Th 2 to a Th1 Response," *Immunology* 109 (2003): 407–14.

18. J. Rehman et al., "Increased Production of Antigen Specific Immunoglobulins G and

M in Vivo Treatment with the Medicinal Plants *Echinacea angustifolia* and *Hydrastis canadensis*," *Immunology Letters* 68 (1999): 391–95.

19. J. Bardy, N.J. Slevin, K.L. Mais, and A. Molassiotis, "A Systematic Review of Honey Uses and Its Potential Values Within Oncology Care," *Journal of Clinical Nursing* 17 (2008): 2604–23.

20. M. Fukuda et al., "Jungle Honey Enhances Immune Function and Antitumor Activity," *Evidence-Based Complementary and Alternative Medicine* (2009); Jan 12 [electronic publication ahead of print].

21. Roxas and Jurenka, "Colds and Influenza," 25–48.

22. No authors listed. "*Glycyrrhiza glabra* monograph," *Alternative Medicine Review* 10 (2005): 230–37; J.H. Dai et al., "Glycyrrhizin Enhances Interleukin-12 Production in Peritoneal Macrophages," *Immunology* 103 (2001): 235–43.

23. T. Utsunomiya et al., "Glycyrrhizin an Active Component of Licorice Roots Reduces Morbidity and Mortality of Mice with Lethal Doses of Influenza Virus," *Antimicrobial Agents and Chemotherapy* 41 (1997): 551–56.

24. Roxas and Jurenka, "Colds and Influenza," 25–48.

25. T. Inoue, Y. Sugimoto, H. Masuda, and C. Kamei, "Effects of Peppermint (*Mentha piperita L*) Extract on Experimental Allergic Rhinitis in Rats," *Biological and Pharmaceutical Bulletin* 24 (2001): 92–5.

26. A. Patenkovic et al., "Antimutagenic Effect of Sage Tea in the Wing Spot Test of *Drosophila melanogaster*," *Food and Chemical Toxicology* 47 (2009): 180–83.

27. S. Buechi et al., "Open Trial Assesses Aspects of Safety and Efficacy of a Combined Herbal Cough Syrup with Ivy and Thyme," *Forsch Komplementarmed Klass Naturheilkd* 12 (2005): 28–332.

Chapter 5: Homeopathic Remedies: Relatively Safe Alternative Medicine

1. I. Loudon, "A Brief History of Homeopathy," *Journal of the Royal Society of Medicine* 99 (2006): 607–10.

2. A. Campbell, "The Origins of Classical Homeopathy?" *Complementary Therapies in Medicine* 7 (1999): 76–82.

3. B. Leary, "The Homeopathic Management of Cholera in the Nineteenth Century with Special Reference to the Epidemic in London in 1854," *Medizine Gesellschaft Geschichte* 16 (1997): 125–44.

4. Loudon, "Brief History of Homeopathy," 607–10.

5. D. Eskinazi, "Homeopathy Re-Visited," *Archives of Internal Medicine* 159 (1999): 1981–87.

6. W.C. Merrell and E. Shalts, "Homeopathy," *Medical Clinics in North America* 86 (2002): 47–62.

7. Eskinazi, "Homeopathy Re-Visited," 1981–87.

8. Loudon, "Brief History of Homeopathy," 607–10.

9. P. Tedesco and J. Cicchetti, "Like Cures Like: Homeopathy," *American Journal of Nursing* 101 (2001): 43–49.

10. Ibid.

11. Loudon, "Brief History of Homeopathy," 607–10.

12. Tedesco and Cicchetti, "Like Cures Like," 43–49.

13. Loudon, "Brief History of Homeopathy," 607–10.

14. Ibid.

15. W.B. Jonas, T. Kaptchuck, and K. Linde, "A Critical View of Homeopathy," *Annals of Internal Medicine* 138 (2003): 393–99.

16. C. Lee, "Homeopathy in Cancer Care Part II: Continuing the Practice of Like Curing Like," *Clinical Journal of Oncology Nursing* 8 (2004): 327–30.

17. Ibid.

18. "Homeopathy: Real Medicine or Empty Promises?" FDA website at http://www.fda.gov/fdac/096_home.html. Accessed 11 February 2009.

19. D. McGraw, "Flu Symptoms? Try Duck; Why Sales of Homeopathic Products Are Soaring Today," *US News and World Report* 122 (1997): 51–52.

20. "Homeopathy: Real Medicine."

21. W.C. Merrell and E. Shalts, "Homeopathy," *Medical Clinics of North America* 86 (2002): 47–62.

22. C. Bayley, "Homeopathy," *Journal of Medical Philosophy* 18 (1993): 129–45.

23. Jonas, Kaptchuk, and Linde, "A Critical Overview," 393–99.

24. Loudon, "Brief History of Homeopathy," 607–10.

25. M.B. Rise and A. Steinsbeck, "How Do Parents of Child Patients Compare Consultations with Homeopaths and Physicians? A Qualitative Study," *Patient Education and Counseling* 74 (2009): 91–96.

26. A.P. Bikker, S.W. Mercer, and D. Reilly, "A Pilot Prospective Study on the Consultation and Rational Empathy: A Patient Enablement and Health Changes Over 12 Months in Patients Going to Glasgow Homeopathic Hospital," *Journal of Alternative and Complementary Medicine* 11 (2005): 591–600.

27. C. Sonnex, "Empathy: Improving the Quality of Genitourinary Medicine Consultation," *International Journal of STD & AIDS* 19 (2008): 73–76.

28. D.J. Anick, "High Sensitivity 1H-NMR Spectroscopy of Homeopathic Remedies Made in Water," *BMC Complementary and Alternative Medicine* 4 (2004): 15.

29. L.R. Milgrom, "A New Geometrical Description of Entanglement and the Curative Homeopathic Process," *Journal of Alternative and Complementary Medicine* 14 (2008): 329–39.

30. Tedesco and Cicchetti, "Like Cures Like," 43–49.

31. M. Stollberg, "Inventing the Randomized Double-Blind Trial: The Nuremberg Salt Test of 1835," *Journal of the Royal Society of Medicine* 99 (2006): 643–44.

32. A. Shang et al., "Are the Clinical Effects of Homeopathy Placebo Effects? Comparative Study of Placebo-Controlled Trials of Homeopathy and Allopathy," *Lancet* 366, no. 9487 (2005): 726–32.

33. A. Paris et al., "Effect of Homeopathy on Analgesic Intake Following Knee Ligament Reconstruction: A Phase III Mono Center Randomized Placebo-Controlled Study," *British Journal of Clinical Pharmacology* 65 (2008): 180–87.

34. C.M. Witt, R. Ludtke, R. Baur, and S.N. Willich, "Homeopathy Medical Practice: Long-Term Results of a Cohort Study With 3981 Patients," *BMC Public Health* 5 (2005): 115.

35. T. Keli, "Homeopathic Versus Conventional Treatment of Children with Eczema: A Comparative Study," *Complementary and Thereutic Medicine* 16 (2008): 15–21.
36. Jonas, Kaptchuk, and Linde, "A Critical Overview," 393–99.
37. J. Kleijnen, P. Knipschild, and G. ter Riet, "Clinical Trial of Homeopathy," *British Medical Journal* 302 (1991): 316–23.
38. M. Weiser, W. Stosser, and P. Klein, "Homeopathic vs Conventional Treatment of Vertigo: A Randomized Double-Blind Controlled Clinical Study," *Archives of Otolaryngology—Head & Neck Surgery* 124 (1998): 879–85.
39. I.R. Bell et al., "Improved Clinical Status in Fibromyalgia Patients Treated with Individualized Homeopathic Remedies versus Placebo," *Rheumatology* (Oxford) 43 (2004): 577–82.
40. Tedesco and Cicchetti, "Like Cures Like," 43–49.
41. J. Lazarou, B.H. Pomeranz, and P.N. Corey, "Incidence of Adverse Drug Reactions in Hospitalized Patients: A Meta Analysis," *Journal of the American Medical Association* 279 (1998): 1200–1205.
42. D. Chakraborti et al., "Arsenic Toxicity from Homeopathic Treatment," *Journal of Toxicology: Clinical Toxicology* 41 (2003): 963–67.

Chapter 6: Vitamins and Minerals

1. C.L. Rock, "Multivitamin-MultiMineral Supplements: Who Uses Them?" *American Journal of Clinical Nutrition* 85 (2007): 277S–279S.
2. P.B. Massey, "Dietary Supplements," *Medical Clinics of North America* 86 (2002): 127–47.
3. K.L. Penniston and S.A. Tanumihardjo, "The Acute and Chronic Toxic Effects of Vitamin A," *American Journal of Clinical Nutrition* 71 (2006): 1325S–1233S.
4. L.C. Heap, T.J. Peters, and S. Wessely, "Vitamin B Status in Patients with Chronic Fatigue Syndrome," *Journal of the Royal Society of Medicine* 92 (1999): 183–85.
5. A. E Beaudin and P.J. Stover, "Insights into Metabolic Mechanisms Underlying Folate Responsive Neural Tube Defects: A Mini Review," *Birth Defects Research Part A Clinical and Molecular Teratology* 2009 January 29 [electronic publication ahead of print].
6. J. Selhub, "Public Health Significances of Elevated Homocysteine," *Food and Nutrition Bulletin* 29, suppl. 2 (2008): 116–25.
7. M. Ebbing et al., "Mortality and Cardiovascular Events in Patients Treated with Homocysteine-Lowering B Vitamins after Coronary Angiography: A Randomized Controlled Trial," *Journal of the American Medical Association* 3000 (2008): 795–804.
8. J.D. Spence, "Homocysteine-Lowering Therapy: A Role in Stroke Prevention," *Lancet Neurology* 6 (2007): 830–38.
9. E. Giovannucci et al., "Multivitamin Use of Folate, and Colon Cancer in Women in the Nurses Health Study," *Annals of Internal Medicine* 129 (1998): 517–24.
10. U. Ericson et al., "High Folate Intake Is Associated with Lower Breast Cancer Incidence in Postmenopausal Women in the Malmö Diet and Cancer Cohort," *American Journal of Nutrition* 86 (2007): 434–43.
11. V. Ganji and M.R. Kafai, "Trends in Serum Folate, RBC Folate, and Circulating

Total Homocysteine Concentrations in the United States: Analysis of Data from National Health and Nutrition Examination Surveys, 1988–1994, 1990–2000 and 2001–2002," *Journal of Nutrition* 136 (2006): 153–58.

12. H. Hemila, "Vitamin C Supplementation and the Common Cold: Was Linus Pauling Right or Wrong?" *International Journal for Vitamin and Nutrition Research* 67 (1997): 329–35.

13. R.M. Douglas and H. Hemila, "Vitamin C for Preventing and Treating Common Cold," *Cochrane Database Systematic Review* 4 (2004): CD000980.

14. H. Hemila, "Vitamin C Supplementation and Respiratory Infections: A Systematic Review," *Military Medicine* 169 (2004): 920–25.

15. R.M. Douglas, H. Hemila, E. Chalker, and B. Tracey, "Vitamin C for Preventing and Treating Common Cold," *Cochrane Database Systematic Review* 3 (2007): CD000980.

16. T.W. Anderson, "Large Scale Studies with Vitamin C," *Acta Vitaminology and Enzymology* 31 (1977): 43–50.

17. H.A. Bischoff-Ferrari et al., "Fracture Prevention with Vitamin D Supplementation: A Meta-Analysis of Randomized Clinical Trials," *Journal of the American Medical Association* 293 (2005): 2257–2264.

18. M.F. Holick and T.C. Chen, "Vitamin D Deficiency: A Worldwide Problem with Health Consequences," *American Journal of Clinical Nutrition* 87 (2008): 1080S–1986S.

19. M.S. Calvo, S.J. Whiting, and C.N. Barton, "Vitamin D Intake: A Global Perspective of Current Status," *Journal of Nutrition* 135 (2005): 310–16.

20. U. Milman et al., "Vitamin E Supplementation Reduces Cardiovascular Events in a Sub-Group Middle-Aged Individuals with Both Type 2 Diabetes and Haptoglobin 2-2 Genotype," *Arteriosclerosis and Thrombosis Vascular Biology* 28 (2008): 341–47.

21. D. Faskanich et al., "Vitamin K Intake and Hip Fractures in Women: A Prospective Study," *American Journal of Clinical Nutrition* 69 (1999): 74–79.

22. E.R. Miller IIIrd et al., "Meta-Analysis: High-Dosage Vitamin E Supplementation May Increase All-Cause Mortality," *Annals of Internal Medicine* 142 (2005): 37–46.

23. G. Bjelakovic et al., "Mortality in Randomized Trials of Antioxidant Supplements for Primary and Secondary Prevention: A Systematic Review and Meta-Analysis," *Journal of the American Medical Association* 297 (2007): 842–857.

24. Y. Zhang et al., "Vitamin and Mineral Use and Risk of Prostate Cancer: The Case-Control Surveillance Study," *Cancer Causes Control* 20 (2009): 691–98.

25. H.C. Lukaski, "Magnesium, Zinc and Chromium Nutriture and Physical Activity," *American Journal of Clinical Nutrition* 72, suppl. 2 (2000): 585–93.

26. J.P. Bonjour et al., "Inhibition of Bone Turnover by Milk Intake in Postmenopausal Women," *British Journal of Nutrition* 100 (2008): 866–74.

27. A. Devine, J.M. Hodgson, I.M. Dick, and R.L. Prince, "Tea Drinking Associated with Benefits on Bone Density in Older Women," *American Journal of Clinical Nutrition* 86 (2007): 1243–47.

28. K. Radimer et al., "Dietary Supplement Use by the U.S. Adults: Data from the National Health and Nutrition Examination Survey, 1999–2000," *American Journal of Epidemiology* 160 (2004): 339–49.

29. W. Hermann and J. Geisel, "Vegetarian Diet and Monitoring of Vitamin B-12 Status," *Clinica Chimica Acta* 326 (2002): 47–59.

30. S.P. Murphy et al., "Multivitamin–Multimineral Supplements' Effect on Total Nutrient Intake," *American Journal of Clinical Nutrition* 85 (2007): S280–84.

31. U. Shaikh, R.S. Byrd, and P. Auinger, "Vitamin and Mineral Supplement Use by the Children and Adolescents in the 1999–2004 National Health and Nutrition Examination Survey: Relationship with Nutrition, Food, Security, Physical Activity and Health Care Access," *Archives of Pediatrics & Adolescent Medicine* 163 (2009): 150–57.

32. R. Briefel et al., "Feeding Infants and Toddlers Study: Do Vitamin and Mineral Supplements Contribute to Nutrient Adequacy or Excess Among U.S. Infants and Toddlers," *Journal of the American Dietetic Association* 106, suppl. 1 (2006): S52–S56.

33. H.Y. Huang et al., "The Efficacy and Safety of Multivitamin and Mineral Supplement Use to Prevent Cancer and Chronic Disease in Adults: A Systematic Review for a National Institutes of Health State of the Science Conference. *Annals of Internal Medicine* 145 (2006): 372–385.

34. M.L. Neuhouser et al., "Multivitamin Use and Risk of Cancer and Cardiovascular Disease in Women's Health Initiative Cohorts," *Archives of Internal Medicine* 169 (2009): 294–304.

Chapter 7: Moderately Toxic Herbal Remedies
That May Cause Organ Damage

1. T. Kawaguchi et al., "Severe Hepatotoxicity Associated with a N-Nitrosofenfluramine-Containing Weight-Loss Product," *Journal of Gastroenterology and Hepatology* 19 (2004): 349–50.

2. L.B. Seeff, "Herbal Hepatotoxicity," *Clinics in Liver Disease* 11 (2007): 577–96.

3. B.C. Nisbet and R.E. O'Connor, "Black Cohosh Induced Hepatitis," *Delaware Medical Journal* 79 (2007): 441–44.

4. G. B Mahady et al., "United States Pharmacopeia Review of the Black Cohosh Case Reports of Hepatotoxicity," *Menopause* 15 (2008): 628–38.

5. S. Alderman et al., "Cholestatic Hepatitis After Ingestion of Chaparral Leaves: Confirmation by Endoscopic Retrograde Cholangiopancreatography and Liver Biopsy," *Journal of Clinical Gastroenterology* 19 (1994): 242–47.

6. N.M. Sheikh, R.M. Philen, and L.A. Love, "Chaparral-Associated Hepatotoxicity," *Archives of Internal Medicine* 157 (1997): 913–19.

7. L. Stickel and H.K. Seitz, "The Efficacy and Safety of Comfrey," *Public Health and Nutrition* 3(4A) (2000): 501–08.

8. A. Castot and D. Larrey, "Hepatitis Observed During a Treatment with a Drug or Tea Containing Wild Germander: Evaluation of 26 Cases Reported to the Regional Centers for Pharmacovigilance," *Clinical Biology* 16 (1992): 916–99 [article in French].

9. L. Laliberte and J.P. Villeneuve, "Hepatitis After Use of Germander, a Herbal Remedy," *Canadian Medical Association Journal* 154 (1996): 1689–92.

10. Seeff, "Herbal Hepatotoxicity," 577–596.

11. D.D. Jamieson, P.H. Duffield, D. Cheng, and A.M. Duffield, "Composition of Cen-

tral Nervous System Activity of the Aqueous and Lipid Extract of Kava (*Piper Methysticum*)," *Archive of International Pharmacodynamics and Therapeutics* 301 (1989): 66–80.

12. J. Scherer, "Kava-Kava Extract in Anxiety Disorders: An Outpatient Observational Study," *Advances in Therapy* 15 (1998): 261–69.

13. U. Jappe, I. Frankle, D. Reinhold, and H.P. Gollnick, "Sebotrophic Drug Reaction Resulting from Kava-Kava Extract Therapy: A New Entity?" *Journal of the American Academy of Dermatology* 38 (1998): 104–06.

14. J.C. Almedi and E.W. Grimsley, "Coma from the Health Food Store: Interaction Between Kava and Alprazolam," *Annals of Internal Medicine* 125 (1996): 940–41.

15. M. Escher and J. Desmeules, "Hepatitis Associated with Kava, an Herbal Remedy," *British Medical Journal* 322 (2001): 139.

16. D.L. Clouatre, "Kava Kava: Examining New Reports of Toxicity," *Toxicology Letters* 150 (2004): 85–96.

17. A. Denham, M.A. McIntyre, and J. Whitehouse, "Kava—The Unfolding Story: Report on a Work-in-Progress," *Journal of Alternative and Complementary Medicine* 8 (2002): 237–63.

18. P.A. Whitton et al., "Kava Lactones and Kava Kava Controversy," *Phytochemistry* 64 (2003): 673–79.

19. J.T. Favreau et al., "Severe Hepatotoxicity Associated with Use of Dietary Supplement," *Annals of Internal Medicine* 136 (2002): 590–95.

20. S. Chitturi and G.C. Farrell, "Hepatotoxic Slimming Aids and Other Herbal Hepatotoxins," *Journal of Gastroenterology and Hepatology* 23 (2008): 355–73.

21. Ibid.

22. J. Harvey and D.G. Colin-Jones, "Mistletoe Hepatitis," *British Medical Journal* (*Clinical Research Edition*) 282, no. 6259 (1981): 186–87.

23. Seeff, "Herbal Hepatotoxicity," 577–596.

24. I.B. Anderson et al., "Pennyroyal Toxicity: Measurement of Toxic Metabolites Levels in Two Cases and Review of Literature," *Annals of Internal Medicine* 124 (1996): 726–34.

25. M. Vanhaelen et al., "Rapidly Progressive Interstitial Renal Fibrosis in Young Women: Association with Slimming Regimen Including Chinese Herb," *Lancet* 341 (1993): 387–91.

26. J. Jellin et al, "Pharmacist's Letter/Prescriber's Letter," Natural Medicines Comprehensive Database, 4th ed. (Stockton, CA: Therapeutic Research Faculty, 2002).

27. M.J. Myhre, "Herbal Remedies, Nephropathies, and Renal Disease," *Nephrology Nursing Journal* 27 (2000): 473–78.

28. E. Ernst, "Cardiovascular Adverse Effects of Herbal Medicines: A Systematic Review of the Recent Literature," *Canadian Journal of Cardiology* 19 (2003): 818–27.

29. Y. Wang et al., "Characterization of Metabolites and Cytochrome P 450 Isoforms Involved in the Microsomal Metabolism of Aconite," *Journal of Chromatography B* 844 (2006): 292–300.

30. R. Pullela et al., "A Case of Fetal Aconite Poisoning by Monkshood," *Journal of Forensic Science* 53 (2008): 491–94.

31. T. Harada et al., "Congestive Heart Failure Caused by Digitalis Toxicity in an Elderly Man Taking Licorice-Containing Chinese Herbal Medicine," *Cardiology* 98 (2002): 218.

32. S. Shilo and H.J. Hirsch, "Iodine-Induced Hyperthyroidism in a Patient with a Normal Thyroid Gland," *Postgraduate Medical Journal* 62 (1996): 661–62.

33. K. Mussig et al., "Iodine-Induced Thyrotoxicosis After Ingestion of Kelp-Containing Tea," *Journal of General Internal Medicine* 21 (2006): C11–14.

Chapter 8: Severely Toxic Herbal Remedies That May Even Cause Death

1. No author listed, "Dangerous Supplements Still at Large," *Consumer Reports* 69 (2004): 12–17.

2. P.P. But, Y.T. Tai, and K. Young, "Three Fatal Cases of Herbal Aconite Poisoning," *Veterinary and Human Toxicology* 36 (1994): 212–15.

3. T.Y. Chan et al., "A Case of Acute Aconite Poisoning Caused by Chuanwu and Caowu," *Journal of Tropical Medical Hygiene* 96 (1993): 62–63.

4. R. Pullela et al., "A Case of Fatal Aconitine Poisoning by Monkshood Ingestion," *Journal of Forensic Science* 53 (2008): 491–94.

5. S. Morishita et al., "Pharmacological Actions of 'Kyushin,' A Drug Containing Toad Venom: Cardiotonic and Arrhythmogenic Effects and Excitatory Effect on Respiration," *American Journal of Chinese Medicine* 20 (1992): 245–46.

6. R. Ko et al., "Lethal Ingestion of Chinese Tea Containing Chan Su," *Western Journal of Medicine* 164 (1996): 71–75.

7. A. Dasgupta et al., "The Fab Fragment of Anti-Digoxin Antibody (Digibind) Binds Digitoxin-like Immunoreactive Components of Chinese Medicine Chan Su: Monitoring the Effect by Measuring the Effects by Measuring Free Digitoxin," *Clinica Chimica Acta* 309 (2001): 91–95.

8. T.L. Barry, G. Petzinger, and S.W. Zito. "GC/MS Comparison of the West Indian Aphrodisiac 'Love Stone' in the Chinese Medicine Chan Su: Bufotenine and Related Bufadienolides," *Journal of Forensic Science* 41 (1996): 1068–73.

9. C.A. Haller and N.L. Benowitz, "Adverse and Central Nervous System Events Associated with Dietary Supplements Containing Ephedra Alkaloids," *New England Journal of Medicine* 343 (2000): 1833–38.

10. M.J. Seamon and K.A. Clauson, "Ephedra: Yesterday, DSHEA, and Tomorrow—A Ten Year Perspective on the Dietary Supplement Health and Education Act of 1994," *Journal of Herbal Pharmacotherapy* 5 (2005): 67–86.

11. F. Stickel, G. Egerer, and H.K. Seitz, "Hepatotoxicity of Botanicals," *Public Health and Nutrition* 3 (2000): 113–24.

12. D.W. Gordon et al., "Chaparral Ingestion: The Broadening Spectrum of Liver Injury Caused by Herbal Medications," *Journal of the American Medical Association* 273 (1995): 489–90.

13. P.J. Gow et al., "Fatal Fulminant Hepatic Failure Induced by a Natural Therapy Containing Kava," *Medical Journal of Australia* 178 (2003): 442–43.

14. M.L. Yeong, B. Swinburn, M. Kennedy, and G. Nicholson, "Hepatic Veno-Occlusive Disease Associated with Comfrey Ingestion," *Journal of Gastroenterology and Hepatology* 5 (1990): 211–14.

15. I.B. Anderson et al., "Pennyroyal Toxicity: Measurement of Toxic Metabolite Levels in Two Cases and Review of Literature," *Annals of Internal Medicine* 124 (1996): 726–34.

16. N. Mostefa-Kara et al., "Fatal Hepatitis after Herbal Tea," *Lancet* 340 (1992): 674.

17. M. Johns Cupp, ed., *Toxicology and Clinical Pharmacology of Herbal Products* (Totowa, NJ: Humana Press, 2000).

18. J.E. Davis, "Are One or Two Dangerous? Methyl Salicylate Exposure in Toddlers," *Journal of Emergency Medicine* 32 (2007): 63–69.

19. T.Y. Chan, "Ingestion of Medicated Oils by Adults: The Risk of Severe Salicylate Poisoning Is Related to the Packaging of These Products," *Human and Experimental Toxicology* 21 (2002): 171–74.

20. D. Parker et al., "The Analysis of Methyl Salicylate and Salicylic Acid from Chinese Herbal Medicine Ingestion," *Journal of Analytical Toxicology* 28 (2004): 214–16.

21. P. Morra et al., "Serum Concentrations of Salicylic Acid Following Topically Applied Salicylate Derivatives," *Annals of Pharmacotherapy* 30 (1996): 935–40.

22. P. O'Malley, "Sports Cream and Arthritic Rubs: The Hidden Dangers of Unrecognized Salicylate Toxicity," *Clinical Nurse Specialist* 22 (2008): 6–8.

23. Morra et al., "Serum Concentrations of Salicylic Acid," 935–40.

24. L.M. Blum and F. Reiders, "Oleander Distribution in a Fatality from Rectal and Oral Nerium Oleander Extracts Administration," *Journal of Analytical Toxicology* 82 (1987): 121–122.

25. D. Brewster, "Herbal Poisoning: A Case Report of Fetal Yellow Oleander Poisoning from the Solomon Islands," *Annals of Tropical Paediatrics* 6 (1986): 289–91.

26. B.E. Haynes, H.A. Bessen, and W.D. Wightman, "Oleander Tea: Herbal Draught of Death," *Annals of Emergency Medicine* 14 (1985): 350–53.

27. M. Eddleston et al., "Deaths Due to the Absence of an Affordable Antitoxin for Plant Poisoning," *Lancet* 362 (2000): 1041–44.

28. W.C. Chou, C.C. Wu, P.C. Yang, and Y.T. Lee, "Hypovolemic Shock and Mortality after Ingestion of Tripterygium Wilfordii Hook F: A Case Report," *International Journal of Cardiology* 49 (1995): 173–77.

29. No author listed, "Crackdown on 'Andro' Products," *FDA Consumer* 38 (2004): 26

30. R. Dhar et al., "Cardiovascular Toxicities of Performance Enhancing Substances in Sports," *Mayo Clinic Proceedings* 80 (2005): 1307–15.

31. S. Haaz et al., "*Citrus Aurantium* and Synephrine Alkaloids in the Treatment of Overweight and Obesity: An Update," *Obesity Research* 7 (2006): 79–88.

32. A.M. Hess and D.L. Sullivan, "Potential for Toxicity with Use of Bitter Orange Extract and Guarana for Weight Loss," *Annals of Pharmacotherapy* 39 (2005): 574–75.

33. Hess and Sullivan, "Potential for Toxicity," 574–75.

34. A. Subarnas, Y. Oshima, and Y. Sidik Ohizumi, "An Antidepressant Principle of Lobelia Inflata L," *Journal of Pharmaceutical Sciences* 81 (1992): 620–21.

35. M.B. Forrester, "Nutmeg Intoxication in Texas: 1998–2004," *Human and Experimental Toxicology* 24 (2005): 563–66.

36. U. Stein, H. Greyer, and H. Hentschel, "Nutmeg Poisoning—Report on a Fatal and a Series of Cases Recorded by a Poison Information Center," *Forensic Science International* 118 (2001): 87–90.

37. H. Hallstrom and A. Thuvander, "Toxicological Evaluation of Myristicin," *Natural Toxins* 5 (1997): 186–92.

38. W.H. Lewis and P.R. Smith, "Pokeroot Herbal Tea Poisoning," *Journal of the American Medical Association* 242 (1979): 2759–60.

39. R.F.B. MacGregor et al., "Hepatotoxicity from Herbal Remedies," *British Medical Journal* 299 (1989): 1156–57.

40. S.D. Weisbord, J.B. Soule, P.L. Kimmel, "Poison On Line—Acute Renal Failure Caused by Oil of Wormwood Purchased Through the Internet," *New England Journal of Medicine* 227 (1997): 825–27.

41. E. Ernst and M.H. Pittler, "Yohimbine for Erectile Dysfunction: A Systematic Review and Meta-Analysis of Randomized Clinical Trials," *Journal of Urology* 159 (1998): 433–36

42. V. Dumestre-Toulet et al., "Last Performance with Viagra: Post-Mortem Identification of Sildenafil and Its Metabolites in Biological Specimens Including Hair Sample," *Forensic Science International* 126 (2002): 71–76.

43. No author listed, "Dangerous Supplements Still at Large," *Consumer Reports* 69 (2004): 12–17.

44. No author listed, "Risky Pills: Supplements to Avoid," *Consumer Reports* 73 (2008): 46–49.

Chapter 9: How Herbal Remedies Interact with Your Medicines

1. T. Kupiec and V. Raj, "Fatal Seizures Due to Potential Herb-Drug Interactions with Ginkgo Biloba," *Journal of Analytical Toxicology* 29 (2005): 755–58.

2. A. Sood et al., "Potential for Interaction Between Dietary Supplements and Prescription Medications," *American Journal of Medicine* 121 (2008): 207–11.

3. X.X. Yang et al., "Drug-Herb Interactions: Eliminating Toxicity with Hard Drug Design," *Current Pharmaceutical Design* 12 (2006): 4649–64.

4. Y.M. Di, C.G. Li, C.C. Xue, and S.F. Zhou, "Clinical Drugs that Interact with St. John's Wort and Implication in Drug Development," *Current Pharmaceutical Design* 14 (2008): 1723–42.

5. E. Ernst, "St. John's Wort Supplements Endanger the Success of Organ Transplantation," *Archives of Surgery* 137 (2002): 316–19.

6. D.J. Greenblatt and L.L. von Moltke, "Interaction of Warfarin with Drugs, Natural Substances and Food," *Journal of Clinical Pharmacology* 45 (2005): 127–32.

7. S. Zhou, E. Chan, E.Q. Pan, M. Huang, and E.J. Lee, "Pharmacokinetic Interactions of Drugs with St. John's Wort," *Journal of Psychopharmacology* 18 (2004): 262–76.

8. Y.N. Singh, "Potential Interaction Between Kava and St. John's Wort," *Journal of Ethnopharmacology* 100 (2005): 108–13.

9. T.O. Cheng, "Not Only Green Tea but Also Green Leafy Vegetables Inhibit Warfarin," [letter], *International Journal of Cardiology* 125 (2008): 101.

10. D.J. Greenblatt and L.L. von Motke, "Interaction of Warfarin with Drugs, Natural Substances and Food," *Journal of Clinical Pharmacology* 45 (2005): 127–32.

11. O. Q.Yin, B. Tomlinson, M.M. Waye, A.H. Chow, and M.S. Chow, "Pharmacoge-

netics and Herb-Drug Interactions: Experience with Ginkgo," *Pharmacogenetics* 14 (2004): 841–50.

12. S. Bent, H. Goldberg, A. Padula, and A.L. Avins, "Spontaneous Bleeding Associated with Ginkgo Biloba: A Case Report and Systemic Review of the Literature," *Journal of General Internal Medicine* 20 (2005): 657–61.

13. B.D. Jones and A.M. Runikis, "Interaction of Ginseng with Phenelzine," *Journal of Clinical Psychopharmacology* 3 (1987): 201–2.

14. L.G. Miller, "Herbal Medicinals: Selected Clinical Considerations Focusing on Known or Potential Drug-Herb Interactions," *Archives of Internal Medicine* 158 (1998): 2200–11.

15. J.C. Almeida, and E.W. Grimsley, "Coma from the Health Food Store: Interaction Between Kava and Alprazolam," *Annals of Internal Medicine* 125, no. 11 (1996): 940–1.

16. C. Dalla-Corte et al., "Potentially Adverse Interactions Between Haloperidol and Valerian," *Food Chemistry and Toxicology* 46 (2008): 2369–75.

17. Miller, "Herbal Medicinals," 2200–11.

18. Ibid.

19. A. Dasgupta, "Herbal Supplements and Therapeutic Drug Monitoring: Focus on Digoxin Immunoassays and Interaction with St. John's Wort," *Therapeutic Drug Monitoring* 30 (2008): 212–17.

Chapter 10: Food, Alcohol, Fruit Juices, Smoking—and Your Meds

1. K. Fujita, "Food Drug Interactions via Human Cytochrome P450 3A (CYP3A)," *Drug Metabolism and Drug Interactions* 20 (2004): 195–217.

2. T.C. Fegan et al., "Increased Clearance of Propranolol and Theophylline by High-Protein Compared with High-Carbohydrate Diet," *Clinical Pharmacology & Therapeutics* 41 (1987): 402–6.

3. D. Genser, "Food and Drug Interaction: Consequences for the Nutrition/Health Status," *Annals of Nutrition and Metabolism* 52, suppl. 1 (2008): 29–32.

4. S. Jordan, H. Griffiths, and R. Griffith, "Administration of Medicines. Part 2. Pharmacology," *Nursing Standard* 18 (2003): 45–54.

5. W. Marcason, "What Is the Bottom Line for Dietary Guidelines when Taking Monoamine Oxidase Inhibitors?" *Journal of the American Dietary Association* 105 (2005): 163.

6. R. Weathermon and D.W. Crabb, "Alcohol and Medication Interactions," *Alcohol Health and Research World* 23 (1999): 40–54.

7. LB Seeff et al. "Acetaminophen Hepatotoxicity in Alcoholics: A Therapeutic Misadventure," *Annals of Internal Medicine* 104 (1986): 399–404.

8. F.T. Wootton and W.M. Lee, "Acetaminophen Hepatotoxicity in the Alcoholic," *South Medical Journal* 89 (1990): 1047–49.

9. Weathermon and Crabb, "Alcohol and Medication Interactions," 40–54.

10. E.V. Hersh, A. Pinto, and P.A. Moore, "Adverse Drug Interactions Involving Common Prescription and Over-the-Counter Analgesic Agents," *Clinical Therapeutics* 29 (2007): S2477–79.

11. L.A. Kroon, "Drug Interactions and Smoking: Raising Awareness for Acute and Critical Care Provider," *Critical Care Nursing Clinics of North America* 18 (2006): 53–62.

12. Ibid.

13. V.J. Colucci and J.E. Knapp, "Increase in International Normalization Ratio Associated with Smoking Cessation," *Annals of Pharmacotherapy* 35 (2001): 385–86.

14. D.G. Bailey, J.D. Spence, C. Munoz, and J.M. Arnold, "Interaction of Citrus Juices with Felodipine and Nifedipine," *Lancet* 337 (1997): 268–69.

15. M. Saito, M. Hirata-Koizumi, M. Matsumoto, T. Urano, R. Hasegawa, "Undesirable Effects of Citrus Juice on the Pharmacokinetics of Drugs: Focus on Recent Studies," *Drug Safety* 28 (2005): 677–94.

16. T. Uno et al., "Effects of Grapefruit Juice on the Stereoselective Disposition of Nicardipine in Humans: Evidence for Dominant Presystematic Elimination at the Gut Site," *European Journal of Clinical Pharmacology* 56(2006): 643–49.

17. R. Tian et al., "Effects of Grapefruit Juice and Orange Juice on the Intestinal Efflux of P-Glycoprotein Substrates," *Pharmaceutical Research* 19 (2002): 802–9.

18. M.F. Paine, W.W. Widmer, H.L. Hart, and S.N. Pusek, "A Furanocoumarin-Free Grapefruit Juice Establishes Furanocoumarins as the Mediators of the Grapefruit Juice–Felodipine Interaction," *American Journal of Clinical Nutrition* 83 (2006): 1097–1105.

19. U. Lundahl, G.C. Regardh, B. Edger, and G. Johnsson, "The Interaction Effect of Grapefruit Juice Is Maximal After the First Glass," *European Journal of Clinical Pharmacology* 54 (1998): 75–81.

20. A. Dahan and H. Altman, "Food-Drug Interaction: Grapefruit Juice Augments Drug Bioavailability-Mechanism, Extent and Relevance," *European Journal of Clinical Nutrition* 58 (2004): 1–9.

21. C. Bistrup, F.T. Nielsen, U.E. Jeppesen, and H. Dieperink, "Effect of Grapefruit Juice on Sandimmune Neoral Absorption Among Stable Renal Allograft Recipients," *Nephrology Dialysis Transplantation* 16 (2001): 373–77.

22. Ibid.; D. Williams and J. Feely, "Pharmacokinetic and Pharmacodynamic Drug Interactions with HMG-COA Reductase Inhibitors," *Clinical Pharmacokinetics* 41 (2002): 432–438.

23. Dahan and Altman, "Food-Drug Interaction," 1–9.

24. P.E. Johnston and A. Milstone, "Probable Interaction of Bergamotting and Cyclosporine in a Lung Transplant Recipient," [Letter to the editor] *Transplantation* 27 (2005): 746.

25. S. Fukatsu et al., "Delayed Effect of Grapefruit Juice on Pharmacokinetics and Pharmacodynamics of Tacrolimus in a Living Donor Transplant Recipient," *Drug Metabolism and Pharmacokinetics* 21 (2006): 122–25.

26. S.K. Garg, N. Kumar, V.K. Bhargava, and S.K. Prabhakar, "Effect of Grapefruit Juice on Carbamazepine Bioavailability in Patients with Epilepsy," *Clinical Pharmacology & Therapeutics* 64 (1998): 286–88.

27. N. Kumar, S.K. Garg, and S. Prabhakar, "Lack of Pharmacokinetic Interaction Between Grapefruit Juice and Phenytoin in Healthy Male Volunteers and Epileptic Pa-

tients," *Methods and Findings in Experimental and Clinical Pharmacology* 21 (1999): 629–32.

28. A. Jetter et al., "Effect of Grapefruit Juice on the Pharmacokinetics of Sildenafil," *Clinical Pharmacology & Therapeutics* 71 (2002): 21–29.

29. Dahan and Altman, "Food-Drug Interaction," 1–9.

30. J.D. Spencer, "Drug Interaction with Grapefruit Juice: Whose Responsibility Is It to Warn the Public?" *Clinical Pharmacology & Therapeutics* 61 (1997): 395–400.

31. G.K. Dresser, R.B. Kim, and D.G. Bailey, "Effect of Grapefruit Juice Volume on the Reduction of Fexofenadine Bioavailability: Possible Role of Anion Transporting Polypeptides," *Clinical Pharmacology & Therapeutics* 77 (2005): 170–77.

32. H.H. Kupferschmidt, K.E. Fattinger, H.R. Ha, F. Follath, and S. Krahenbuhl, "Grapefruit Juice Enhances the Bioavailability of HIV Protease Inhibitor Saquinavir in Man," *British Journal of Clinical Pharmacology* 45 (1998): 355–59.

33. D. Demarles et al., "Single Dose Pharmacokinetics of Amprenavir Co-administered with Grapefruit Juice," *Antimicrobial Agents and Chemotherapy* 46 (2002): 1589–90.

34. S.R. Penzak et al., "Effect of Seville Orange Juice and Grapefruit Juice on Indinavir Pharmacokinetics," *Journal of Clinical Pharmacology* 42 (2002): 1165–70.

35. Dahan and Altman, "Food-Drug Interaction," 1–9.

36. S. Malhotra, D.G. Bailey, M.F. Paine, and P. B.Watkins, "Seville Orange Juice–Felodipine Interaction: Comparison with Dilute Grapefruit Juice and Involvement of Furocoumarins," *Clinical Pharmacology & Therapeutics* 69 (2001): 14–23.

37. J.J. Lilja, L. Juntti-Patinen, and P.J. Neuvonen, "Orange Juice Substantially Reduced the Bioavailability of the Beta-Adrenergic Blocking Agent Celiprolol," *Clinical Pharmacology & Therapeutics* 75 (2004): 184–90.

38. D.E. Nix, et al., "Pharmacokinetics and Relative Bioavailability of Clofazimine in Relation to Food, Orange Juice and Antacid," *Tuberculosis* (Edinburgh) 84 (2004): 365–73.

39. Y. Koitabashi et al., "Orange Juice Increased Bioavailability of Pravastatin, 3-Hydroxy-3-Methylglutaryl CoA Reductase Inhibitor in Rats and Healthy Human Subjects," *Life Sciences* 78 (2006): 2852–59.

40. J. Grenier et al., "Pomelo Juice but Not Cranberry Juice Affects the Pharmacokinetics of Cyclosporine in Humans," *Clinical Pharmacology & Therapeutics* 79 (2006): 255–62.

41. Ibid.

42. R. Suvarna, M. Pirmohamed, and L. Henderson, "Possible Interaction between Warfarin and Cranberry Juice," *British Medical Journal* 327 (2003): 1454.

43. A.V. Sorokin, B. Duncan, R. Panetta, and P.D. Thompson, "Rhabdomyolysis Associated with Pomegranate Juice Consumption," *American Journal of Cardiology* 98 (2006): 705–6.

Chapter 11: Herbal Supplements, Alternative Therapies, and Women's Health

1. S.E. Geller and L. Studee, "Botanical and Dietary Supplements for Menopausal Symptoms: What Works and What Does Not," *Journal of Women's Health* 14 (2005): 634–49.

2. E. Ernst, "Herbal Medicinal Plants During Pregnancy: Are They Safe?" *BJOG: An International Journal of Obstetrics and Gynecology* 109 (2002): 227–35.

3. D.M. Marcus and W.R. Snodgrass, "Do No Harm: Avoidance of Herbal Medicines During Pregnancy," *Obstetrics and Gynecology* 105 (2005): 1119–22.

4. Ernst, "Herbal Medicinal Plants," 227–35.

5. J.J. Dugoua et al., "Safety and Efficacy of Blue Cohosh (*Caulophyllum thalictroides*) During Pregnancy and Lactation," *Canadian Journal of Clinical Pharmacology* 15 (2008): e66–73.

6. D.R. Gardner et al., "Abortifacient Effects of Lodgepole Pine (*Pinus contorta*) and Common Juniper (*Juniperus communis*) on Cattle," *Veterinary and Human Toxicology* 40 (1998): 260–63.

7. J.J. Dugoua et al., "Safety and Efficacy of Black Cohosh (*Cimicifuga racemosa*) During Pregnancy and Lactation," *Canadian Journal of Clinical Pharmacology* 13 (2006): e257–61.

8. C. Ciganda and A. Laborde, "Herbal Infusions Used for Induced Abortion," *Journal of Toxicology: Clinical Toxicology* 41 (2003): 235–39.

9. Ernst, "Herbal Medicinal Plants," 227–35.

10. M. Gallo et al., "Pregnancy Outcome Following Gestational Exposure to Echinacea: A Prospective Controlled Study," *Archives of Internal Medicine* 160 (2000): 3141–43.

11. J.J. Dugoua et al., "Safety and Efficacy of Cranberry (*Vaccinium macrocarpon*) During Pregnancy and Lactation," *Canadian Journal of Clinical Pharmacology* 15 (2008): e80–86.

12. J. Ensiyeh and M.A. Sakineh, "Comparing Ginger and Vitamin B6 for the Treatment of Nausea and Vomiting in Pregnancy: A Randomised Controlled Trial," *Midwifery* 25 (2009): 649–53.

13. F. Borrelli et al., "Effectiveness and Safety of Ginger in the Treatment of Pregnancy Related Nausea and Vomiting," *Obstetrics and Gynecology* 105 (2005): 849–56.

14. W. Wuttke et al., "Chaste Tree (*Vitex agnus-castus*) Pharmacology and Clinical Indications," *Phytomedicine* 10 (2003): 348–57.

15. B.C. Lucks, J. Sorensen, and L. Veal, "Vitex Agnus-Castus Essential Oil and Menopausal Balance: A Self-Care Survey," *Complementary Therapy Nursing Midwifery* 8 (2002): 148–54.

16. C. Daniele et al., "Vitex Agnus-Castus: A Systematic Review of Adverse Events," *Drug Safety* 28 (2005): 319–32.

17. R.G. Jepson and J.C. Craig, "A Systematic Review of the Evidence for Cranberries and Blueberries in UTI Prevention," *Molecular Nutrition & Food Research* 51 (2007): 738–45.

18. M.J. Hess et al. "Evaluation of Cranberry Tablets for the Prevention of Urinary Tract Infections in Spinal Cord Injured Patients with Neurogenic Bladder," *Spinal Cord* 46 (2008): 622–26.

19. M.E. McMurdo et al., "Cranberry or Trimethoprim for the Prevention of Recurrent Urinary Tract Infection? A Randomized Controlled Clinical Trial in Older Women," *Journal of Antimicrobial Chemotherapy* 63 (2009): 389–95.

20. I. T. Lee et al., "Effect of Cranberry Extract on Lipid Profiles in Subjects with Type 2 Diabetes," *Diabetic Medicine* 25 (2008): 1473–77.

21. No author listed, "Monograph *Angelica sinensis*," *Alternative Medicine Review* 9 (2004): 429–33.

22. C. J. Haines et al., "A Randomized, Double-Blind, Placebo-Controlled Study of the Effect of a Chinese Herbal Medicine Preparation (Dang Gui Buxue Tang) on Menopausal Symptoms in Hong Kong Chinese Women," *Climateric* 11 (2008): 244–51.

23. A. Heyerick et al., "A First Perspective Randomized, Double-Blind Placebo-Controlled Study on the Use of a Standardized Hop Extract to Alleviate Menopausal Discomforts," *Maturitas* 54 (2006): 164–75.

24. T. Low Dog, "Menopause: A Review of Botanical Dietary Supplements," *American Journal of Medicine* 118 (2005): 98S–108S.

25. P. B. Clifton-Bligh et al., "The Effect of Isoflavones Extracted from Red Clover (Rimostil) on Lipid and Bone Metabolism," *Menopause* 8 (2001): 259–65.

26. Low Dog, "Menopause: A Review," 98S–108S.

27. Ibid.

28. E. A. Nahas et al., "Efficacy and Safety of a Soy Isoflavone Extract in Postmenopausal Women: A Randomized Double-Blind and Placebo-Controlled Study," *Maturitas* 58 (2007): 249–58.

29. A. Atmaca et al., "Soy Isoflavone in the Management of Postmenopausal Osteoporosis," *Menopause* 15 (2008): 748–57.

30. Low Dog, "Menopause: A Review," 98S–108S.

31. Ibid.

32. P. A. Komesaroff et al., "Effects of Wild Yam Extract on Menopausal Symptoms, Lipids and Sex Hormones in Healthy Menopausal Women," *Climacteric* 4 (2001): 144–50.

33. R. Uebelhack et al., "Black Cohosh and St. John's Wort for Climacteric Complaints: A Randomized Trial," *Obstetrics and Gynecology* 107 (2006): 247–55.

34. A. V. Patel, J. Rojas-Vera, and C. G. Dacke, "Therapeutic Constituents and Actions of Rubes Species," *Current Medicinal Chemistry* 11 (2004): 1501–12.

35. M. Parson, M. Simpson, and T. Ponton, "Raspberry Leaf and Its Effect on Labor: Safety and Efficacy," *Australian College of Midwives Inc. Journal* 12 (1999): 20–25.

36. M. Simpson et al., "Raspberry Leaf in Pregnancy: Its Safety and Efficacy in Labor," *Journal of Midwifery Women's Health* 46 (2001): 51–59.

37. Y. Nir et al., "Acupuncture for Postmenopausal Hot Flashes," *Maturitas* 56 (2007): 389–95.

38. S. Murakami et al., "Aromatherapy for Outpatients with Menopausal Symptoms in Obstetrics and Gynecology," *Journal of Alternative and Complementary Medicine* 11 (2005): 491–94.

39. C. A. Smith et al., "Complementary and Alternative Therapies for Pain Management in Labour," *Cochrane Database Systematic Review* 18 (2006): CD003521.

40. O. Can Gurkan and H. Arslan, "Effect of Acupressure on Nausea and Vomiting During Pregnancy," *Complementary Therapies in Clinical Practice* 14 (2008): 46–52.

Chapter 12: How Herbal Remedies May Affect Laboratory Test Results

1. E.L. Archer and D.K. Boyle, "Herb and Supplement Use Among the Retail Population of an Independent Urban Herb Store," *Journal of Holistic Nursing* 26 (2008): 27–35.

2. M. Escher et al., "Hepatitis Associated with Kava, a Herbal Remedy for Anxiety," *British Medical Journal* 322 (2001): 139.

3. G. Millonig, S. Stadlmann, and W. Vogel, "Herbal Hepatotoxicity: Acute Hepatitis Caused by a Noni Preparation (*Morinda citrifolia*)," *European Journal of Gasteroenterology and Hepatology* 17 (2005): 445–47.

4. A.M. Karch and F.E. Jarch, "The Herb Garden. Remember to Ask Your Patients All About Preparations," *American Journal of Nursing* 99 (1999): 12.

5. S.P. Bunner and R. McGinnis, "Chromium-Induced Hypoglycemia," [Letter to the editor], *Psychosomatics* 39 (1998): 298–99

6. G.Y. Yeh, et al., "Systematic Review of Herbs and Dietary Supplements for Glycemic Control in Diabetes," *Diabetes Care* 26 (2003): 1277–94.

7. Bunner and McGinnis, "Chromium-Induced Hypoglycemia," 298–99.

8. Ibid.

9. A. Serraclara et al., "Hypoglycemic Action of an Oral Fig Leaf Decoction in Type 1 Diabetic Patients," *Diabetes Research and Clinical Practice* 39 (1998): 19–22.

10. R. Iida et al., "Pseudoaldosteronism Due to the Concurrent Use of Two Herbal Medicines Containing Glycyrrhizin: Interaction of Glycyrrhizin with Angiotensin-Converting Enzyme Inhibitor," *Clinical and Experimental Nephrology* 10 (2006): 131–135.

11. S.M. Ahmed, N.R. Banner, and S.W. Dubrey, "Low Cyclosporine-A Level Due to Saint-John's-Wort in Heart Transplant Patients," *Journal of Heart and Lung Transplant* 20 (2001): 795.

12. S. McRae, "Elevated Serum Digoxin Levels in a Patient Taking Digoxin and Siberian Ginseng," *Canadian Medical Association Journal* 155 (1996): 293–95.

13. A. Dasgupta et al., "Positive and Negative Interference of Chinese Medicine Chan Su in Serum Digoxin Measurement: Elimination of Interference by Using a Monoclonal Chemiluminescent Digoxin Assay or Monitoring Free Digoxin Concentration," *American Journal of Clinical Pathology* 114 (2000): 174–179.

14. A.D. Kaye, I. Kucera, and R. Saber, "Perioperative Anesthesia Clinical Consideration of Alternative Medicines," *Anesthesiology Clinics of North America* 22 (2004): 125–39.

15. M. Ang-Lee, J. Moss, and C.S. Yuan, "Herbal Medicines and Perioperative Care," *Journal of the American Medical Association* 286 (2001): 208–16.

16. Kaye, Kucera, and Saber, "Perioperative Anesthesia Clinical Consideration," 125–39.

17. A. Dasgupta and D.W. Bernard, "Complementary and Alternative Medicines: Effects on Clinical Laboratory Tests," *Archives of Pathology and Laboratory Medicine* 130 (2006): 521–28.

Chapter 13: Herbal Remedies Misidentified or Contaminated with Heavy Metals or Western Drugs

1. P.A. Routledge, "The European Herbal Medicine Directives: Could It Have Saved the Lives of Romeo and Juliet?" *Drug Safety* 31 (2008): 416–18.
2. R.J. Huxtable, "The Harmful Potential of Herbal and Other Plant Products," *Drug Safety* 5 (1990): S126–36.
3. N. Slifman et al., "Contamination of Botanical Dietary Supplements by Digitalis Lantana," *New England Journal of Medicine* 339 (1998): 806–10.
4. A. Dasgupta, B. Davis, and A. Wells, "Effect of Plantain on Therapeutic Drug Monitoring of Digoxin and Thirteen Other Common Drugs," *Annals of Clinial Biochemistry* 43 (2006): 223–35.
5. G. Koren et al., "Maternal Use of Ginseng and Neonatal Androgenization," *Journal of the American Medical Association* 264 (1990): 2866.
6. A.J. Turley and D.F. Muir, "ECG for Physicians: A Potentially Fatal Case of Mistaken Identity," *Resuscitation* 76 (2008): 323–24.
7. M. Madhok et al., "*Amanita bisporigera* Ingestion: Mistaken Identity, Dose-Related Toxicity and Improvement Despite Severe Toxicity," *Pediatric Emergency Care* 22 (2006): 177–80.
8. B.L. O'Brien and U. Khuu, "A Fatal Sunday Brunch: Amanita Mushroom Poisoning in a Gulf Coast Family," *American Journal of Gastroenterology* 91 (1996): 581–83.
9. H.R. Petty et al., "Identification of Colchicine in Placental Blood from Patients Using Herbal Medicines," *Chemical Research and Toxicology* 14 (2001): 1254–58.
10. R.B. Saper et al., "Lead, Mercury and Arsenic in U.S. and Indian Manufactured Ayurvedic Medicines Sold via the Internet," *Journal of the American Medical Association* 300 (2008): 915–23.
11. E.D. Caldas and L.L. Machado, "Cadmium, Mercury and Lead in Medicinal Herbs in Brazil," *Food and Chemical Toxicology* 42 (2004): 599–603.
12. K. Cooper et al., "Public Health Risks From Heavy Metals and Metalloids Present in Traditional Chinese Medicines," *Journal of Toxicology and Environmental Health A* 70 (2007): 1694–99.
13. E. Obi et al., "Heavy Metal Hazards of Nigerian Herbal Supplements," *Science of the Total Environment* 369 (2006): 35–41.
14. G.J. Gravey et al., "Heavy Metal Hazards of Asian Traditional Medicines," *International Journal of Environmental Health Research* 11 (2001): 63–71.
15. S. Lowenberg, "Scientists Tackle Water Contamination in Bangladesh," *Lancet* 370, no. 9586 (2007): 471–72.
16. N. Singh, D. Jumar, and A.P. Sahu, "Arsenic in the Environment: Effects on Human Health and Possible Prevention," *Journal of Environmental Biology* 28, suppl. 2 (2007): 359–65.
17. E. Amster, A. Tiwary, and M.B. Schenker, "Case Report: Potential Arsenic Toxicosis Secondary to Herbal Kelp Supplement," *Environmental Health Perspectives* 115 (2007): 606–08.
18. S.B. Markowitz et al., "Lead Poisoning Due to Hai Ge Fen: The Porphyrin Content

of Individual Erythrocytes," *Journal of the American Medical Association* 271 (1994): 932–34.

19. J. Barthwal, S. Nair, and P. Kakkar, "Heavy Metal Accumulation in Medicinal Plants Collected from Environmentally Different Sites," *Biomedial and Environmental Sciences* 21 (2008): 319–24.

20. J. Xue, L. Hao, and F. Peng, "Residues of 18 Organochlorine Pesticides in 30 Traditional Chinese Medicines," *Chemosphere* 71 (2008): 1051–55.

21. K.S. Leung et al., "Systematic Evaluation of Organochlorine Pesticide Residue in Chinese Materia Medica," *Phytotherapy Research* 19 (2005): 514–18.

22. M. J Hsieh et al., "Acute Cholinergic Syndrome Following Ingestion of Contaminated Herbal Extract," *Emergency Medicine Journal* 25 (2008): 781–82.

23. W. F Huang, K.C. Wen, and M.L. Hsiao, "Adulteration by Synthetic Therapeutic Substances of Traditional Chinese Medicine in Taiwan," *Journal of Clinical Pharmacology* 37 (1997): 344–50.

24. K.K. Lau, C.K. Lai, and A.Y.W. Chan, "Phenytoin Poisoning after Using Chinese Proprietary Medicines," *Human and Experimental Toxicology* 19 (2000): 385–86.

25. P.L. Eachus, "Positive Drug Screen for Benzodiazepine Due to a Chinese Herbal Product," *Journal of Athletic Training* 31 (1996): 165–66.

26. M.H. Nguyen et al., "Amphetamine Lacing of an Internet Marketed Nutraceutical," *Mayo Clinic Proceedings* 81 (2006): 1627–29.

27. A.M. Goudie and J.M. Kaye, "Contaminated Medication Precipitating Hypoglycemia," *Medical Journal of Australia* 175 (2001): 256–57.

28. G. Lau et al., "A Fatal Case of Hepatic Failure Possibly Induced by Nitrosofenfluramine: A Case Report," *Medicine, Science and the Law* 44 (2004): 252–63.

29. Y.R. Ku et al., "Analysis of Synthetic Anti-Diabetic Drugs in Adulterated Traditional Chinese Medicines by High Performance Capillary Electrophoresis," *Journal of Pharmaceutical and Biomedical Analysis* 33 (2003): 329–34.

30. Y.R. Ku et al., "Analysis and Confirmation of Synthetic Anorexics in Adulterated Traditional Chinese Medicines by High Capillary Electrophoresis," *Journal of Chromatography* A 848 (1999): 537–43.

31. L. Nelson, R. Shih, and R. Hoffman, "Aplastic Anemia Induced by an Adulterated Herbal Medication," *Journal of Toxicology: Clinical Toxicology* 33 (1995): 467–70.

32. C.K. Wang et al., "Anti HIV Cyclotides from Chinese Medicinal Herb Viola Yedoensis," *Journal of Natural Products* 71 (2008): 47–52.

33. E. Ernst, "Adulteration of Chinese Herbal Medicines with Synthetic Drugs: A Systematic Review," *Journal of Internal Medicine* 252 (2002): 107–13.

Chapter 14: An Introduction to Ayurvedic Medicine

1. B.B. Aggarwal et al., "Curcumin: The Indian Solid Gold," *Advances in Experimental Medicine and Biology* 595 (2007): 1–75.

2. A. Narayanasamy and M. Narayanasamy, "Ayurveda Medicine: An Introduction for Nurses," *British Journal of Nursing* 15 (2006): 1185–90.

3. R. Mamtani and R. Mamtani, "Ayurveda and Yoga in Cardiovascular Diseases," *Cardiology in Review* 13 (2005): 155–62.

4. Ibid.

5. A. Chopra and V.V. Doiphode, "Ayurvedic Medicine Core-Concept, Therapeutic Principles and Current Relevance," *Medical Clinics of North America* 86 (2002): 75–88.

6. Aggarwal et al., "Curcumin," 1–75.

7. J.M. Ringman et al., "A Potential Role of the Curry Spice Curcumin in Alzheimer's Disease," *Current Alzheimer Research* 2 (2005): 131–36.

8. P. Prakash and N. Gupta, "Therapeutic Use of *Ocimum Sanctum* (Tulsi) with a Note on Eugenol and Its Pharmacological Actions: A Short Review," *Indian Journal of Physiology and Pharmacology* 49 (2005): 125–31.

9. R. Subapriya and S. Naginin, "Medicinal Properties of Neem Leaves: A Review," *Current Medicinal Chemistry and Anticancer Agents* 5 (2005): 149–56

10. R.H. Singh, K. Narisimhamurthy, and G. Singh, "Neuro Nutrient Impact of Ayurvedic Rasayana Therapy in Brain Aging," *Biogerontology* 9 (2008): 369–74.

11. L.A. Norh, L.B. Rasmussen, and J. Strand, "Resin from the Mukul Myrrh Tree, Guggul, Can It Be Used for Treating Hypercholesterolemia? A Randomized Controlled Study," *Complementary Therapies in Medicine* 17 (2009): 16–22.

12. A. Vaidya and T. Devasagayam, "Current Status of Herbal Drugs in India: An Overview," *Journal of Clinical Biochemistry and Nutrition* 41 (2007): 1–11.

13. A. Kumar et al., "Bhasmas: Unique Ayurvedic Metallic-Herbal Preparations, Chemical Characterization," *Biological Trace Element Research* 109 (2006): 231–54.

14. D.V. Datta et al., "Chronic Oral Arsenic Intoxication as a Possible Etiological Factor in Idiopathic Portal Hypertension (Non-Cirrhotic Portal Fibrosis) in India," *Gut* 20 (1979): 378–84.

15. Ibid.

16. R.B. Saper et al., "Heavy Metal Content of Ayurvedic Herbal Medicine Products," *Journal of the American Medical Association* 292 (2004): 2868–73.

17. R.B. Saper et al., "Lead, Mercury and Arsenic in US- and Indian-Manufactured Ayurvedic Medicines Sold via the Internet," *Journal of the American Medical Association* 300 (2008): 915–23.

18. Ibid.

19. Centers for Disease Control and Prevention (CDC), "Lead Poisoning Associated with Ayurvedic Medications—Five States, 2000–2003," *MMWR Morbidity and Mortality Weekly Report* 53 (2004): 582–84.

20. S.N. Kales, C.A. Christophi, and R.B. Saper, "Hematopoietic Toxicity from Lead-Containing Ayurvedic Medications," *Medical Science Monitor* 13 (2007): CR295–98.

21. B.M. Spriewald et al., "Lead Induced Anaemia Due to Traditional Indian Medicine: A Case Report," *Occupational and Environmental Medicine* 56 (1999): 282–83.

22. M.G. von Vonderen et al., "Severe Gastrointestinal Symptoms Due to Lead Poisoning from Indian Traditional Medicine," *American Journal of Gastroenterology* 95 (2000): 1591–92.

23. P.A. Tait et al., "Severe Congenital Lead Poisoning in a Preterm Infant Due to a Herbal Remedy," *Medical Journal of Australia* 177 (2002): 193–95.

24. S. Khandpur et al., "Chronic Arsenic Toxicity from Ayurvedic Medicines," *International Journal of Dermatology* 47 (2008): 618–21.
25. Saper et al., "Lead, Mercury and Arsenic," 915–23.
26. S. Singh and M. Kumar, "Heavy Metal Load of Soil, Water and Vegetables in Peri-Urban Delhi," *Environmental Monitoring and Assessment* 120 (2006): 79–91.

Glossary

antibody: An antibody is a specific protein belonging to a class of molecules known as immunoglobulins. Antibodies are produced by the body's immune system when a foreign object such as a bacteria, parasite, or virus invades the body. Antibodies then identify and, if possible, neutralize the invading foreign object by binding with the object.

antigen: An antigen is a foreign object that can cause the body's immune system to react. An antigen can simply be pollen which stimulates immune system to cause allergy, but it can also be a bacteria, virus, or parasite that stimulates the body's immune system to fight back by producing antibodies.

blood electrolyte: Blood electrolytes are various positively charged and negatively charged atoms (ions) that are essential components of all living organisms. Major electrolytes found in blood are collectively referred to as blood electrolytes. These ions include sodium, potassium, magnesium, chloride, bicarbonate, phosphate, and sulfate. Imbalances of electrolytes can cause serious illness, including death.

blood sugar/blood glucose: Blood sugar, also referred to as blood glucose, is the concentration of glucose in serum, which is the water part of blood. A normal concentration of blood glucose is 70–99 mg in 100 mL of blood.

cardiovascular disease: Cardiac means "heart" and vascular means "blood vessels." Therefore, cardiovascular disease is collectively various diseases of heart and blood vessels related to the blood supply of the heart. Heart attack, medically termed as myocardial infarction, is a common type of heart disease that occurs when the blood supply to the heart is severely impaired due to blockage of one or more of the arteries that supply blood to the heart. In addition, abnormal heart rhythms (arrhythmias), heart block (see below), heart failure, and congenital defects of the heart can also be classified under cardiovascular diseases, which are the number-one killer in the world, claiming millions of lives every year.

cytochrome P-450: Cytochrome P-450 comprises a large family of over fifty different iron-containing enzymes that collectively act as the body's largest detoxification system. These enzymes convert many harmful substances and drugs into more water-soluble forms so that these substances can be readily excreted in the urine. In addition, many other compounds produced by our body (endogenous compounds), such as various hormones, are also transformed into more soluble forms by these enzymes.

drug metabolism: Metabolism of a drug is a chemical transformation process by which a drug molecule is converted into a more water-soluble form so that the body can get rid of a drug through excretion into the urine. The cytochrome P-450 family of enzymes is responsible for the metabolism of a large number of drugs. In addition, various other enzymes are also present in the liver; for example, uranidine-5-diphos-phoglucuronosyltransferase. Some drugs may undergo minimal metabolism and may be excreted through the bile into feces.

heart block: Heart block is a disease in which there is a blockage of the electrical conduction system in the heart. This is different from heart attack, in which the blood supply to the heart is impaired due to blockage in one or more arteries.

heavy metals: Heavy metals is a loosely defined term which refers to metallic compounds that have toxicity. Most commonly, these metals are lead, mercury, arsenic, cadmium and chromium, although other metals also have known toxicity, such as the light metal beryllium.

heme: Heme is the nonprotein part of hemoglobin that contains iron.

hepatocyte: Hepatocytes are the major cell type found in the liver, and they perform many important functions in the liver, including producing many proteins, degrading carbohydrates, producing clotting factors of the blood, and detoxifying the body by transforming drugs and toxic substances into a more water-soluble form for excretion in the urine.

hormone replacement therapy: Hormone replacement therapy (HRT), sometimes also referred as estrogen replacement therapy, is used to supplement estrogen and sometimes progesterone (progestin, a synthetic form is also used) in women undergoing menopause in order to alleviate menopausal symptoms. HRT must be carefully monitored by a physician because this therapy may also increase risks of breast cancer, heart disease, and stroke.

hypoglycemia: Hypoglycemia is a condition in which the concentration of blood glucose is significantly lower than 70 mg per 100 mL of blood, the lower end of normal blood glucose level. Symptoms of hypoglycemia are nonspecific, ranging from not feeling good, to lightheadedness, to sweating, and even to becoming unconscious. Usually symptoms are found in people with blood glucose below 55 mg per 100 mL of blood. Hypoglycemia may arise in a diabetic patient due to therapy complications.

immunoassay: An immunoassay is a biochemical test that uses specific proteins called antibodies to measure the concentration of a substance—a drug or another protein—in biological liquids like blood and urine.

intestinal motility: Intestinal muscle contraction.

lactose: Lactose is a sugar found in milk.

liver enzymes: Enzymes are proteins that catalyze (accelerate) various chemical reactions essential for living organisms. Liver enzymes are enzymes that are found in high amounts in the liver, and in case of liver disease these enzymes are found in higher amounts in the blood through biochemical tests that measure these enzymes, which are known as liver-function tests. Four liver enzymes are commonly measured to investigate liver disease. These enzymes include aspartate aminotransferase (AST), alanine aminotransferase (AST), alkaline phosphatase (ALT), and gamma-glutamyltransferase (GGT).

lymphocytes: Lymphocytes are white blood cells that play major functions in the body's immune system. There are two major types of lymphocytes. B-cells produce antibodies, while T-cells attach harmful cells such as cells infected by a virus or cancer cells.

hepatotoxic: Drugs or other compounds that are toxic to the liver.

macrophage: A macrophage ("big eater" in Greek) is a type of large white blood cell that engulfs and digests pathogens; for example, a harmful bacteria and cellular debris. Macrophages play an important role in the body's immune function.

marker: A marker is a substance found in a large amount in an organ but in a very small amount in the blood. When an organ is damaged, this compound may be released into the blood and can be detected by a laboratory test.

mast cells: Mast cells are also a part of the body's immune system, but these cells are not circulated in the blood; rather, they are bound to various tissues throughout the body. Exact functions of mast cells are not well understood, but they play an important role in defense against the invasion of a harmful parasite. Mast cells are full of histamine, a chemical that is released during the cell's activation, causing allergic reaction.

P-glycoprotein (efflux transporter): P-glycoprotein, also referred as PGP, is a protein that belongs to a large family of proteins that are found in the gut, kidneys, brain, and other organs. These proteins act as an efflux transporter (pump), they transport certain substances from circulation back into the gut, and they also transport substances out of the brain and into the urine or bile, thus helping the body to rid itself of harmful foreign substances. In tumors that are resistant to drugs, these glycoproteins are found on the surface of the tumor cells, and their function is to pump drugs out of tumor cells. Unfortunately, as a result, a tumor may not respond to chemotherapy.

pharmacodynamic interaction: Pharmacodynamic interaction occurs when one drug increases or decreases the action of another drug without altering its level in the blood. For example, drinking alcohol is not recommend if you take a sleeping pill such as diazepam (valium) because alcohol can increase the drowsiness caused by valium by further depressing the central nervous system.

pharmacokinetic interaction: When the movement of one drug in the body through the process of absorption from the gut, distribution in various tissues, degradation (metabolism) by the liver, and excretion from the body is affected by another drug, the interaction is called "pharmacokinetic interaction." Such interaction may increase or decrease the blood level of a drug. For example, one heart medication, quinidine, increases the blood level of another heart medication, digoxin, by pharmacokinetic interaction, thus causing digoxin toxicity. Therefore, a physician reduces dosage of digoxin if quinidine is added to the therapy of a patient.

phytoestrogens: Phytoestrogens are complex compounds that are found in various plants and have some structural similarity with the female hormone estrogen. Phytoestrogens are also referred as dietary estrogens. For example, soy is a source of phytoestrogens.

prosthetic group (heme): A prosthetic group is a nonprotein part of a complex protein. Heme is an iron-containing complex molecule that is the prosthetic group of hemoglobin responsible for carrying oxygen in the blood.

serotonin syndrome: Serotonin is a chemical produced by the body that is required for proper function of nerve cells in the brain. Serotonin syndrome occurs when excess serotonin accumulates in nerves due to increased dosage of an antidepressant such as fluoxetine (Prozac) or when a new antidepressant is added to the regimen of current antidepressants. Many other drugs can cause serotonin syndrome and, in the case of an overdose caused by an antidepressant or an illicit drug, serotonin syndrome may be potentially life-threatening, requiring immediate medical intervention.

Further Reading

Aronson, Jeffrey K. *Meyler's Side Effects of Herbal Medicines*. San Diego, CA: Elsevier Science, 2009.

Arrowsmith, Nancy. *Essential Herbal Wisdom: A Complete Exploration of 50 Remarkable Herbs*. Woodbury, MN: Llewellyn Publications, 2009.

Brown, Donald J. *Herbal Prescriptions for Health & Healing: Your Everyday Guide to Using Herbs Safely and Effectively*. 2nd ed. Twin Lakes, WI: Lotus Press, 2003.

Kane, Charles. *Herbal Medicine: Trends and Traditions (A Comprehensive Sourcebook on the Preparation and Use of Medicinal Plants)*. Oracle, AZ: Lincoln Town Press, 2009.

McIntyre, Anne. *Herbal Treatment of Children: Western and Ayurvedic Perspective*. Woburn, MA: Butterworth-Heinemann, 2005.

Mukherjee, Pulok K., and Peter J. Hougton, eds. *Evaluation of Herbal Medicine Products: Perspectives on Quality, Safety and Efficacy*. London: Pharmaceutical Press, 2009.

Nolan, Linda, and Lyle E. Craker. *Herbs, Spices, and Medicinal Plants*. Oxford, U.K.: Routledge, 2010.

Ramawat, K.G., ed. *Herbal Drugs: Ethnomedicine to Modern Medicine*. New York: Springer, 2009.

Scheid, Volker, Dan Bensky, Andrew Ellis, and Randall Baronet, eds, trans. *Chinese Herbal Medicine: Formulas & Strategies*. 2nd ed. Seattle, WA: Eastland Press, 2009.

Ulbricht, Catherine, and Erica Seamon. *Natural Standard Herbal Pharmacotherapy: An Evidence-Based Approach*. Philadelphia, PA: Mosby, 2009.

Wichtl, Max, ed. *Herbal Drugs and Phytopharmaceuticals*. 3rd ed. Stuttgart, Germany: Medpharm, 2004.

Willamson, Elizabeth, Samuel Driver, and Karen Baxter. *Stockley's Herbal Medicines Interactions: A Guide to the Interactions of Herbal Medicines, Dietary Supplements and Nutraceuticals with Conventional Medicines*. London: Pharmaceutical Press, 2009.

Index